Mass Mediated Disease

Mass Mediated Disease

A Case Study Analysis of Three Flu Pandemics and Public Health Policy

Debra E. Blakely

LEXINGTON BOOKS

A division of
ROWMAN & LITTLEFIELD PUBLISHERS, INC.
Lanham • Boulder • New York • Toronto • Oxford

LEXINGTON BOOKS

A division of Rowman & Littlefield Publishers, Inc.
A wholly owned subsidiary of The Rowman & Littlefield Publishing Group, Inc.
4501 Forbes Boulevard, Suite 200
Lanham, MD 20706

PO Box 317
Oxford
OX2 9RU, UK

British Library Cataloguing in Publication Information Available

Library of Congress Cataloging-in-Publication Data

Blakely, Debra Ellen Menconi.
Mass mediated disease : a case study analysis of three flu pandemics and public health policy / Debra E. Blakely.
p. cm.
Includes bibliographical references and index.
ISBN-13: 978-0-7391-1387-5 (cloth : alk. paper)
ISBN-10: 0-7391-1387-9 (cloth : alk. paper)
1. Influenza—Press coverage—Case studies. 2. Epidemics—Press coverage—Case studies. 3. Influenza—History—20th century—Case studies. 4. Epidemics—History—20th century—Case studies. 5. Mass media in health education—Case studies. I. Title.
RC150.4.B53 2006
616.2'03—dc22 2006003952

Printed in the United States of America

™ The paper used in this publication meets the minimum requirements of American National Standard for Information Sciences—Permanence of Paper for Printed Library Materials, ANSI/NISO Z39.48–1992.

Contents

Acknowledgments

I would like to thank my family, friends, and colleagues for their support, advice, and patience. A heartfelt thanks to Britney, Trey, Simone, Terri, Deborah, Arbie, Patrick, Nilesh, and Jerry.

I would also like to acknowledge the reader. Thank you for taking the time to read though this text. Hopefully you will develop an appreciation for the journalists who help provide some insight into the world around us. While the media are often criticized, their role in presenting facts offers us all an opportunity to learn more about our past and stay connected to our present. I hope this monograph helps to give some insight into how we can critically assess media coverage and use this information to remedy the future.

INTRODUCTION

Infectious diseases have had a profound effect on human history from the Black Death in the fourteenth and sixteenth centuries, cholera in the nineteenth century, flu in the early twentieth century, to AIDS and hepatitis in our own time. Infectious diseases are part of human social systems:[1] the concept of disease is always a social and historical product of culture, and most people now develop such concepts through mass media.[2] Their sense of reality, drawn as it is from cultural artifacts such as newspapers and television, is socially constructed.[3] Just as language is a social and historical product of culture, so, too, is the concept of disease.[4] So, if we wish to understand how we are affected by concepts of disease, we must examine the media's role in articulating those concepts. The purpose of this book is to represent the social construction of disease in the twentieth century, showing how it changed during the century, and how it affected public health policy.

In trying to understand how a public constructed a given disease at a given time we must turn to the constructs themselves, the mediated news stories.[5] These create what some scholars call the "frames" through which people understand their experience, as defined by some overall theme.[6] Accordingly, I have based my conclusions on an analysis of print news stories and editorials about disease in the *New York Times*, *The Times* (London), and popular American magazines.

I chose pandemic influenza as the object of this historical analysis because of its tremendous and continuing impact. In 1918, an influenza pandemic is said to have caused over fifty million deaths worldwide.[7] Since then, each year the flu season has held the possibility of another pandemic; to date, three distinct pandemics have involved the United States, all within the fifty-year time period, 1918–1969. Since medical researchers have not been able to isolate the deadly Spanish influenza virus, or produce a suitable vaccine, it has the potential to resurface with the same lethal destruction as it did in 1918, potentially causing a catastrophic and to-date unimaginable death toll.[8] Currently, the U.S. government has given much attention to pandemic influenza, raising the alarm, again, that a major influenza pandemic is long overdue.

Katherine Anne Porter, who had contracted the disease and survived, wrote a short story, *Pale Horse, Pale Rider* (1936), that gives some insight into the first, Spanish influenza, pandemic.

> "The men are dying like flies out there anyway. This funny new disease. Simply knocks you into a cocked hat."
>
> "It seems to be a plague," said Miranda, "something out of the Middle Ages. Did you ever see so many funerals, ever?"[9]

Later, the flu comes to dominate society:

> "All the theaters and nearly all the shops and restaurants are closed, and the streets have been full of funerals all day and ambulances all night," [Adam said].[10]

Porter's character herself contracts the flu, and reflects:

> The road to death is a long march beset with all evils, and the heart fails little by little at each new terror, the bones rebel at each step, the mind sets up its own bitter resistance and to what end?[11]

To date, scholars have had little to say directly about the social construction of disease; however, there are several useful histories and analyses on related topics—the history of science reporting by the *New York Times*, which had a formative place in the development of science reporting,[12] general histories about influenza, general histories of newspapers that mention disease coverage,[13] specific analyses critiquing reportage on disease, or examining the rhetoric of risk contained in news stories about disease—and to these I will now turn.

HISTORY OF SCIENCE REPORTING THROUGH THE *NEW YORK TIMES*

Much has been written about the importance of reporting about public health issues, or more generally about science reporting,[14] which refers to a broad range of topics, from the physical sciences and the art sciences of medicine and health care, to the application of science through engineering and technology. Science reporting about epidemics and diseases reflects an intense public interest in medical events.[15] In fact, it dates from the inception of the first American newspaper, when *Publik Occurances* in 1690 reported on "epidemical" fevers throughout the colonies (Emery and

Emery, 1988). In reaction the governor of Massachusetts, an early media critic, suppressed further mention of smallpox, and for the moment this reportage simply ended. In 1720, a fiery debate erupted between the editors, James and Benjamin Franklin, of the *New England Courant*, and Cotton Mather, over smallpox and public health concerns in this local paper.[16]

Cushman (1982) and Ziporyn (1988) describe reporting about epidemics in the late nineteenth and early twentieth centuries.[17] Science stories have been available to the *mass* audience since the first mass-produced newspaper in 1834 in New York City. However, during the nineteenth century, such newspapers tended to focus on the bizarre rather than the helpful or useful.[18] The expanding use of newswire services increased the speed of communication and the embarrassment of scientists, whose work was often embellished and sensationalized.[19]

Cassedy (1964) regards the muckraker Samuel Hopkins Adams as laying the groundwork for medical journalism practices that are still in use.[20] Hillman (1965) explains sensationalism in the press as due to *both* journalists reporting out of curiosity and medical scientists presenting information to journalists in exaggerated or sensationalized ways.[21] However this may be, the *New York Times*, which after 1896 established the standard for modern mass-circulation reportage,[22] attempted to steer clear of sensationalized stories throughout the muckraking years and focused instead on reporting factual information.[23] Despite this policy the *Times* thrived, with a circulation of 343,000 by 1920.[24] The *Times* had earned a "badge of respectability" in reporting facts and not sensation.[25]

Though science stories may often have been embellished, systematic social investigation was growing in popularity across all disciplines in this period, and science was becoming a "magical" word in America. Though some reporters thought of themselves as artistic creators of stories, most believed that they should provide facts, and some, a few of whom were trained in science, were given to conceiving journalism in such terms. These reporters helped externalize the idea of science and make it into an American institution.[26] Kovarik (1993/1994), however, points out that despite their concern with scientific objectivity, reporters often fell back on familiar ground, using industry sources rather than objective experts.[27]

During this period Carr Vattel Van Anda became the *New York Times*'s managing editor, a post he held from 1904 until his retirement in 1932. Despite his unpretentious, unassuming nature, Van Anda holds a place as one of the most powerful influences in the history of journalism.[28] He helped to change the face of the modern newspaper. Among his many talents was his skill at comprehending anything scientific.[29] In 1905, Albert Einstein released his theories of relativity, fueling the speculation of reporters and the imagination of the American public; he was covered by *New York Times* reporter Alva Johnston, who went on to win a Pulitzer

Prize for distinguished reporting on scientific news in 1923—all during Van Anda's tenure as editor. On one occasion, Van Anda noticed in a news photo of Albert Einstein that a formula written on a chalkboard in the background was inaccurate. He brought this to the attention of Einstein, who agreed with him.[30]

Between the world wars, a new type of science journalist began to emerge, one who was actually educated in the sciences.[31] Journalists began to move away from both strict factual information and muckraking sensationalism, and toward skepticism and suspicion. These then became ingrained in social thought as a proper approach to anything scientific, as the only way to achieve about it something we would today consider objectivity. This development had, however, been's anticipated by the *New York Times*. Michael Schudson and Meyer Berger both attribute to Adolph S. Ochs of the *Times* the creation of a standard for objective reporting as early as 1896.[32] Joseph Pulitzer, publisher for the *New York Times*'s major competing newspaper, *The World*, once confided to Van Anda in 1904 that he read the *Times* to stay abreast of the news.[33] In 1927 the *New York Times* hired Waldemar Kaempffert to write science editorials. Kaempffert was probably one of the first science editors on any American newspaper.[34]

With the advent of World War II, science gained a new importance for the mass-media audience, which was naturally interested in such matters as nuclear power. Most of the reporting during this time, like most other endeavors, both professional and scientific, was geared toward the war effort.[35] In 1934, only twelve members formed the National Association of Science Writers (NASW).[36] In 1938, only eleven reporters attended the American Association for the Advancement of Sciences (AAAS). Yet in 1942 the *New York Times* hired William L. Laurence as the first newspaper reporter assigned exclusively to science coverage. As early as 1939, Lawrence was reporting about uranium and atomic energy; his terminology on this topic was widely adopted by other reporters. He was the first to report on the atomic bomb dropped on Japan in 1945. When the war ended, the United States Army gave Lawrence permission to give a more complete picture of the development of the atom bomb.[37] With Kaempffert writing news editorials and interpreting science stories, and Lawrence writing science news stories, the *New York Times* held a formative position in science news reporting, and had a head start over other American newspapers.[38] The *New York Times* devoted more news space than any other daily journal to keeping track of America's quest for knowledge and growing preoccupation with anything scientific.[39] This was in part due to Van Anda's influence.[40]

Already in the 1940s the press was subject to increasing suspicion. In 1942, the Hutchins Commission on Freedom of the Press was established to consider press regulations.[41] The most innovative outcome of this Commission was the development of social responsibility theory, which was a call for media to be responsible in fostering productive and creative communities.[42]

By 1951, the *Times*, with 1,350 employees and correspondents in all major cities abroad, was universally recognized as a newspaper of record.[43] Max Frankel, the managing editor for the *New York Times* during and after this period, describes the era as expanding the concept of what news was. During the transition from World War II and the events that led up to the Cold War, the editorial tone of the *New York Times*, though more critical, remained restrained.

According to Schudson, the objectivity debate of the 1960s was a generational debate between those who had fought in World War II and those who were born to the "affluence and anxiety of the Cold War."[44] He claims that the social structure of newsgathering led to a slant in journalism that reinforced official viewpoints of social reality.[45] This was reflected in reporting on McCarthyism, the Cold War, and the Korean War.

These debates about objectivity and increasing concern about news bias led to several new developments in journalism: a rise in interpretive reporting, investigative journalism, creative feature writing techniques, and overall journalistic skepticism. Rosenfeld (1999), in a historical commentary about his personal experience as a science reporter from the 1960s into the 1980s, claims that science reporting evolved from a warning system to an investigative system for the general public.[46] He cites the Tuskegee syphilis study (which broke July 25, 1972) as an example of the results of the current investigative role of the press.

Schudson claims that two conditions made these changes possible: first, an increased presence in government's management of the news since World War II; and second, the adversary culture of the 1960s, which did not trust government and therefore encouraged journalists to be more aggressive. This tension affected science reporting, leading to conflict between scientists who wrote for professional scientific or medical journals, and journalists who wrote science or medical stories for the popular press. The conflict arose in part from sourcing: professional scientists were concerned with cautious accuracy, their claims grounded in empirical data or substantiated by previous literature, while journalists were concerned primarily with newsworthiness. Increased government funding for scientific endeavors set up scientists for the same type of scrutiny as government institutions. These conflicts have attracted scholarly attention and debate.[47]

In the 1960s, new educational programs for science reporters began in earnest at universities and writers' associations. Though scientists, having been ridiculed in the past, and hoping to conceal their work from competitors, were reluctant to release new information about their discoveries and inventions, they were pressured to do so by their professional associations. This was due in part to the insistence of politicians, who were arranging funding through government programs and grants. In 1961, 362 media representatives attended the annual AAAS meeting.[48] During the late 1960s, science reporters captured the American public's attention with accounts of the NASA space program and man's first steps on the moon. By the 1970s, the NASW had 750 members, and the American Medical Writers Association had 1,500.[49] Science reporting was now a well-established beat, with a rich history, and continues to hold a prominent place in news narratives.[50]

INFLUENZA HISTORY

The Centers for Disease Control and Prevention (CDC) define three flu pandemics that have involved the United States: the 1918 Spanish Flu, the 1957 Asian Flu, and the 1968 Hong Kong Flu. However, there is evidence of three previous pandemics involving the United States: in 1650, in 1847, and in 1889.[51] The flu pandemics cover a formative time period for science reporting, and for medical breakthroughs against infectious diseases, one of which came just before the first flu pandemic of 1918. In 1884, Robert Koch first identified the cholera bacillus and thereby opened the door to germ theories and magic bullet cures. Concerned, rich, and well-educated citizens and physicians joined together to create an American agenda for public health, using germ theories to press for improved sanitation.[52]

The influenza virus has been traced to a strain that appeared in Valencia, Spain, in 1650. The Spanish word *influenza,* which means "to influence," was added to the medical lexicon in 1918. Influenza has since been a subject of much speculation and research. Hoehling (1961) describes the influenza as a beautiful but entirely unscrupulous woman, who continues to fascinate men of medicine, though they have so often been hurt by her deadly flirtations. Of course, the quest to identify and unlock the deadly scientific mystery surrounding influenza long preceded the use of the word. In 412 B.C., Hippocrates chronicled an infection that was similar to influenza.[53] Much later, after scientific investigative tools such as the microscope had been invented, a Berlin professor and pathologist, Richard Pfeiffer, isolated a bacterium that he identified as a cause of influenza as early as 1892. In 1918, "Pfeiffer's bacteria" was identified in several influenza victims at Fort Riley, Kansas. Shortly thereafter, and well into the next year, this strain of influenza became known as Spanish influenza and claimed fifty million victims worldwide.

During 1918, much of the world was taken up with a world war; the earliest influenza victims were soldiers stationed in overcrowded camps preparing for war.[54] Hoehling (1961) traces the path of infection and death from Fort Riley in March 1918, to France in May, and to the rest of the world by July. There was, apparently, a five-month span, from March to August, before the first U.S. civilians began contracting the disease and mortality rates began to soar. On August 12, 1918, identified as the day that Americans were hit with the world's deadliest flu virus, the *Bergensfjord,* a Norwegian liner, docked at a Brooklyn, New York, Army base with eleven semiconscious passengers and reports of other victims buried at sea.[55] Within hours of docking, one of the eleven died at a hospital in Brooklyn. From that moment on, illness and death swept the United States for nearly two years. After the 1918 Spanish flu pandemic, and before the next pandemic in 1957, scientists worldwide were on their guard, anticipating the next wave of Spanish influenza. However, the Spanish influenza virus seemed to disappear. The 1957 and 1968 pandemics were not as deadly as the 1918 flu, and neither has received much historical or academic attention.

Since the elimination of smallpox in 1968, the high point for the World Health Organization (WHO), infectious organisms have launched a counteroffensive with resistant strains of malaria, tuberculosis, streptococcus, HIV, and now hepatitis C.[56] Changes in human behavior and modern air travel assure the continuation of an accelerated process of disease homogenization around the world. The flu virus, which evolves a new variant almost every year, is typical of this process.[57] Infectious disease has played and will continue to play a major role in human history, profoundly affecting society in a number of ways. And since the media develop our concepts about disease, and those concepts ultimately affect how we choose to deal with it, media portrayal of disease is well worth examining closely.[58]

ACADEMIC RESEARCH ABOUT INFLUENZA AND SCIENCE REPORTING

There have been few studies of reporting on influenza, and these have been devoted almost exclusively to the 1918 pandemic. A recurrent theme in these studies is the reluctance of journalists to report much, if anything, about the severity of the 1918 flu.[59] Crosby (1989) referred to the 1918 pandemic as the "forgotten pandemic," unimportant because, at the time he performed his research, most scientists believed all major infectious diseases would soon be eliminated.[60] Kolata (1999), a longtime science news reporter for the *New York Times,* reiterated the idea in her book about the 1918 flu pandemic: "The flu's enormous impact somehow escaped attention."[61] She was moved to write by recent stories about the flu that had made it timely again.[62] Scientists, availing themselves of advances in genetic testing and virus identification, had recently discovered pieces of the 1918 flu virus in human remains frozen in the Arctic tundra since 1918, and more in a government warehouse. Both Hume (2000) and Kolata claim that, because of a lack of media coverage during the 1918 pandemic, it was essentially lost to public memory.[63] Another study finds that reporting on the 1918 flu relied heavily on scientific sources, which produced traditional authoritative frames of reference for them.[64] There is also a study of the 1977 Swine Flu Vaccine Program and another of communication strategies for future flu pandemics.[65] No peer-reviewed communication studies address the 1957 or 1968 influenza pandemics.

Several more general studies of science reporting on epidemics and disease have appeared during the last fifty years. According to Krieghbaum (1959) the first public opinion survey results on the subject, in 1957, showed that Americans rely a great deal upon the news media for information about science.[66] Medical stories are most interesting to respondents, especially those about deadly diseases. Schramm (1962) concludes from Krieghbaum's results and another survey performed a year later that science information is widely distributed by media, but the likelihood of readers' comprehending that information depends largely on their educational level.[67] He concludes that the mass media's science agenda does not necessarily benefit those wanting to inform and those being informed.[68] Tannenbaum (1963) combines Krieghbaum's and Schramm's surveys with additional research on communication and science information.[69] He argues that the mass media translate scientific information into terms they deem comprehensible, rather than terms either scientists or the general public deem comprehensible. He reiterates Schramm's claim that the mass media does not necessarily serve those wanting to inform and to be informed about science. Essentially, these early studies reached three general conclusions about science reporting: (1) the media serve as a source of information, (2) the audience may or may not comprehend that information, and (3) the media frame information in science news stories. Generally, science-reporting studies are concerned with at least one of these conclusions.

Added to that, more than six million medical articles are published each year.[70] The public is inundated with medical advice and contrary views from multiple sources, including newspaper stories based on these articles, or on the word of the physicians who read and write them. According to one authoritative analysis, less than 15 percent of all articles published on a particular topic are useful.[71] Studies about science reporting tend to focus on scientists' interaction with the media,[72] or on readers' perceptions of media coverage,[73] or on the public's willingness to rely upon science reporting for medical information,[74] or on the role of media in reporting and framing health-related issues.[75]

In the late 1970s, researchers began to look at science reporting about risk.[76] According to one study, because of changes in social perspectives, science and technology stories increasingly concerned risk.[77] Throughout the 1980s, the management of risk remained an important topic of both theoretical and applied research.[78] A number of studies find that science reporting often presents science or scientists stereotypically as the heroic solution to frightening problems, and that these stereotypes are the result not of the business of journalism, or customary news practices, but of predominant cultural ideas.[79] Another study finds that initial coverage of emerging health risks creates frames that can heighten public anxiety.[80] War metaphors are common, and science stories are structured like morality plays, where the disease is the villain and science the hero.[81]

METHODOLOGY

Reality is socially constructed; critical events can reshape the frames of discourse to produce a conceptual consensus.[82] News stories and editorials provide such frames[83]—the centrally organizing story lines or themes that produce social meaning. Effective analysis of news stories therefore must regard them "both as a body of work that is a continuing story of human activity, and as individual stories that contribute to that continuing one." I have sought to analyze in this manner all *New York Times* items, supplemented by articles from *The Times* (London) and articles accessible through the *Readers' Guide to Periodical Literature* for each pandemic.[84]

First, I examined all available newspaper articles that were identified under the keyword "influenza" by the *New York Times* indexes for each pandemic. Since the flu season begins each fall in October, and runs through March of the next year, I analyzed the calendar years preceding and following the flu pandemic year. For the Spanish influenza, I used the 1917, 1918, 1919, and 1920 indexes. For the 1957 Asian flu, I used the 1957, 1958, 1959, and 1960 indexes, and for the 1969 Asian flu pandemic I used the 1967, 1968, 1969, and 1970 indexes.[85] In total, I examined 835 articles from the *New York Times*, 614 articles from *The Times* (London), and 121 magazine articles. These included news stories, wire stories, correspondent stories, letters to the editor, and editorials.

I chose the *New York Times* because of its elite status. It has a reputation for national and international agenda setting; McCombs has claimed that it can set the agenda as firmly as any president or dictator.[86] When the *New York Times* increases its coverage of a particular topic, most of the nation's other media outlets will follow, devoting prime news time or space to that topic.[87] The *New York Times* has had a consistent index since the mid-nineteenth century. It is thus the best purposive primary source for a study of a public health issue covered by print media over time. Since my purpose is to measure and describe the representation of influenza not over space, from one city to another, but over time, from pandemic to pandemic, I have not made an exhaustive survey of other newspapers.

In order to add depth and breadth to this study, I have incorporated into it coverage from *The Times* (London) and stories indexed by the *Readers' Guide to Periodical Literature*. *The Times* (London) adds an international context and cultural comparison; the indexed magazines reflect the "popular press" in the United States. The *Readers' Guide to Periodical Literature*, which indexes feature articles in U.S. magazines and professional publications, also has a consistent index that covers this time frame (1917–1970). I considered all available articles that appeared under the keyword "influenza" in *Palmer's Index to The Times*, and the *Readers' Guide to Periodical Literature* according to the same system I used with the *New York Times* index: for the year before, the two years during, and the year after the pandemic. However, the *New York Times* remains my primary source.

THEORETICAL ASSUMPTIONS

The idea that we construct our views of reality was originally presented by William James in 1869.[88] In 1935, Kenneth Burke reinforced and extended James's constructionist theories by analyzing narratives as social constructs.[89] Mannheim (1936), building on James's work, represents ideology as a sociology of knowledge that seeks to comprehend thought in a historical-social situation.[90] He claims that every society has special groups of people, "intelligentsia," whose function is to provide an interpretation of the world for that society.[91] Alfred Schultz (1945) reiterates this point, and claims further that multiple realities may be assigned in socially constructing reality itself.[92] Peter L. Berger and Thomas Luckmann (1966) add to this theory by differentiating everyday life from other realities.[93] Goffman (1986) explains that in order to make sense of reality, to understand "what is going on," humans, through discourse, create frames.[94]

Chesebro (1984) explains that this type of social construction is guided by six principles: (1) attention is focused on human constructions or interpretations; (2) the construction is created through symbols; (3) the focus is on socially shared understandings or concepts; (4) social framing is employed, and perspective is a central and unifying critical principle; (5) every socially shared perspective offers one view of truth which can be challenged and contradicted by alternative perspectives of reality; and (6) multiple standards create a self-conscious sense of the potentials and limitations of a symbolically constructed reality.[95]

Tuchman (1978a, b) explains that within the context of socially constructed meaning, reporters, following professional imperatives, use specific methods to create and control controversies. Journalistic professionalism and the structural constraints of daily news work lead news workers to focus on the present and ignore the larger context, or the structure of social action. They prefer to cover events, not issues, and rely on established institutions for information. This limits dissidents' access to media, since their analyses of issues are not properly events and are therefore unworthy of coverage.[96]

The purpose of a framing analysis is to uncover the devices that frame the social construction of reality, the central organizing story lines that provide for social meaning.[97] By defining a group of framing devices, a researcher can understand the conceptual framework through which news texts mediate the history they present.[98] This study will use news stories as a "unified body" of work, with patterns and framing devices that thematically define each pandemic.[99] As the case studies will demonstrate, news stories about influenza make up a continuing story, since influenza is an annual public health threat each winter.

SOURCES OF FRAMES FOR THE CONSTRUCTION OF PANDEMIC DISEASE

Narrative structures—plot conflicts, war metaphors, and the like—can provide media audiences with frames for understanding disease.[100] Controversies, especially those relevant to important themes in American life, can frame pandemic disease as a conflict between competing public interests dealing with a major public health issue.[101] Several recurring frames arise in mediated public health discourse about disease: the importance of the problem, its impact, its cause, and the strength of the evidence of any of these.[102] Some studies have shown that, since arbiters determine the strength of evidence, they should be considered for a framing analysis.[103] Another frame is provided by the public policy outcomes to which disease pandemics may lead.[104] All these frames provide starting points for understanding the construction of pandemic diseases.

Some have claimed that frames can also be provided by contextual devices—such as frequency, placement, visuals, and length of stories—created through news production processes.[105] These processes are, however, as others have shown, themselves subject to predominant cultural ideas about science,[106] and they can distract researchers from the structural qualities of individual stories.[107] I have not therefore employed them explicitly as frames for this study. My focus is not on *how* the narrative is being constructed through news practices, but on *what* is being framed in the stories themselves, in their narrative structure, their use of arbiters, and their concern with public health policy.[108]

As to narrative discourse I examine specifically how in a story the pandemic is defined, how it is imagined as impacting a community, and whether it is conceived in terms involving blame or war. I examine whether, for example, the story emphasizes high mortality rates, since media can compete avidly in stories about medical risks, and as a result, frame them in such a way as to heighten anxiety.[109] News stories often attempt to attribute blame for the disease, since beliefs about responsibility for diseases are central to all cultural understandings of the human condition.[110] Following Davis, I find blame attributed to four general categories: race, immorality, lifestyles, and government or authorities.[111] Previous studies have established that war metaphors are common in science stories; accordingly, I examined pandemic stories for aggressive imagery or metaphors. The metaphors of a science story generally present science as a solution to an intractable problem; I thus consider them carefully in identifying and evaluating the theme of each pandemic.[112]

As to arbiters, I pay close attention to who was providing what information about influenza in the stories, including scientists, medical practitioners, or government authorities.[113]

As to public health policy, media coverage of a health risk can reverberate through the political system, forcing responses from politicians; and media framing can affect public policy.[114] According to Davis, policymakers have four options in shaping health policy: (1) the medical approach, which is to identify and treat the individual; (2) the behavioral approach, which is to try to change a behavior through persuasion, inducement, or coercion; (3) the ecological approach, which is to try to change the disease-promoting environment; or (4) to conduct further research.[115]

In general, through such analysis, I seek to identify an overall theme for each pandemic, to compare these themes, and thus to ascertain whether or not shifts took place over time, and why or why not. Therefore, chapter 2 is a case study analysis of the Spanish Influenza Pandemic of 1918, chapter 3 is a case study analysis of the Asian Influenza Pandemic of 1957, and chapter 4 is a case study analysis of the Hong Kong Influenza Pandemic of 1968. Chapter 5 concludes this text with an overall discussion of each of the frames: narrative discourse, arbiters, and public health policies.

NOTES

1. W. H. McNeill, *Plagues and Peoples*. (New York: Anchor Books, 1998).
2. H. Krieghbaum, "Public Interest in Science News," *Science* 129 (1959): 1092–95; W. Schramm, *Science and the Public Mind* (Stanford: Stanford University

Press for the AAAS, 1962); R. E. Rice and C. Atkin, "Principles of Successful Public Communication Campaigns," in *Media Effects: Advances in Theory and Research*, ed. J. Bryant and D. Zillman (Hillsdale: Lawrence Erlbaum Associates, 1994), 365–88; and T. Ziporyn, *Disease in the Popular American Press: The Case of Diphtheria, Typhoid Fever, and Syphilis, 1870–1920* (New York: Greenwood Press, 1988).

3. P. L. Berger and T. Luckmann, *The Social Construction of Reality: A Treatise in the Sociology of Knowledge* (Garden City, NJ: Doubleday, 1966); G. Tuchman, *Making News: A Study in the Construction of Reality* (New York: Free Press, 1978).

4. McNeill, *Plagues*.

5. J. Hume, "The 'Forgotten' 1918 Influenza Epidemic and Press Portrayal of Public Anxiety," *Journalism and Mass Communication Quarterly* 77 (4) (2000): 898–915; Tuchman, *Making News*.

6. Z. Pan and G. Kosicki, "Framing Analysis: An Approach to News Discourse," *Political Communication* 10 (1993): 55–75.

7. N. F. Cantor, *In The Wake of the Plague: The Black Death and The World It Made* (New York: Free Press, 2001).

8. M. Alvarez and R. Begue, "Eradication of Infectious Diseases: A Goal for the Next Century," Infectious Diseases Society of America (paper presented at Infectious Diseases Society of America Thirty-seventh Annual Meeting, Nov. 20, 1999); G. Kolata, *Flu: The Story of the Great Influenza Pandemic of 1918 and the Search for the Virus that Caused It* (New York: Farrar, Straus and Giroux, 1999); A. Monto, D. Iacuzio, and J. La Montague, "Pandemic Influenza: Confronting a Reemergent Threat," *Journal of Infectious Diseases* 176 (Suppl. 1, 1997): S1–3.

9. K. A. Porter, *Pale Horse, Pale Rider: Three Short Novels* (New York: Modern Library, 1998), 155.

10. Porter, *Pale Horse, Pale Rider*, 181.

11. Porter, *Pale Horse, Pale Rider*, 193.

12. M. Berger, *The Story of the New York Times: 1851–1951* (New York: Simon & Schuster, 1951); B. Fine, *A Giant of the Press* (New York: Editor & Publisher Co., 1933); M. McCombs, "News Influence on Our Pictures of the World," in *Media Effects: Advances in Theory and Research*, 1994): 1–16; and M. Schudson, *Discovering the News: A social history of American newspapers* (New York: Basic Books, 1978), 88–120.

13. See, G. Kolata, *Flu: The story of the great influenza pandemic of 1918 and the search for the virus that caused it* (New York: Farrar, Straus and Giroux, 1999), W. I. B. Beveridge, *Influenza: The Last Great Plague an Unfinished Story* (London: Heinemann, 1977); B. E. Davila, *La Gripe Española. La Pandemica de 1918–1919* (Madrid: Centro de Investigaciones Sociologicas, 1993); A. A. Hoehling, *The Great Epidemic* (Boston: Little, Brown and Co., 1961); K. D. Patterson, *Pandemic Influenza, 1700–1900* (Totowa, NJ: Rowman & Littlefield, 1986); E. Emery and M. Emery, *The Press and America*, 6th ed. (Englewood Cliffs, NJ: Prentice Hall, 1988); and Schudson, *Discovering the News*.

14. L. J. Albrecht, "A Dose of Information: What are Your Patients Reading?" *Texas Medicine* (Sept. 1992): 36–42; C. N. Barnard, "Medicine and the Mass Media," *American Journal of Cardiology* 30 (1972): 579–80; E. V. Boisaubin, "Charity, the Media, and Limited Medical Resources," *JAMA* 259, no. 9 (1988): 1375–76; L. DeBakey, "Medicine and the Press: Resolving Conflicts," *Clinical Research* 22 (1974): 214–25; M. Goldsmith, "Directed to Defend its *Raison d'etre*, NIH Holds Communications Conference," *JAMA* 272, no. 10 (1995): 761–64; I. H. Page, "Science

Writers, Physicians, and the Public—Ménage à Trois," *Annals of Internal Medicine* 73 (1970): 641–47; D. Satcher, "Prescription: Communication," *Quill* 82, no. 9 (1994): 66–67; G. Schwitzer, "Medicine in the Media: The Magical Medical Media Tour," *JAMA* 267, no. 14 (1992): 1969–71; V. de Semir, "What is Newsworthy?" *Lancet* 347 (1996); 1063–66; M. Shuchman and M. S. Wilkes, "Medical Scientists and Health News Reporting: A Case of Miscommunication," Annals of Internal Medicine 126, no. 12 (1997): 976–82; J. Turney, "Public Understanding of Science," *Lancet* 347 (1996): 1087–90; and J. Turrow, "Television Entertainment and the U.S. Health-care Debate," *Lancet* 347 (1996): 1240–43.

15. D. E. Blakely, *Mass Mediated Disease: A Case Study Analysis of News Reporting of Three Influenza Pandemics and Public Health Policy* (Hattiesburg: University of Southern Mississippi, 2001).

16. W. J. Paisley, "Public Communication Campaigns: The American Experience," in *Public Communication Campaigns*, R. E. Rice and W. J. Paisley, eds. (Beverly Hills, CA: Sage, 1981), 15–40.

17. P. Cushman, "Medicine at the Turn of the Century: Perspectives From the Press," New York State Journal of Medicine (1982): 81–84; and Ziporyn, *Disease in the Popular American Press*. Nuwer (1996/1997) used reporting about an 1878 yellow fever epidemic in Mississippi to illustrate how a community dealt with the intense suffering.

18. W. Burkett, *News Reporting: Science, Medicine, and High Technology* (Ames: Iowa State University Press, 1986).

19. Ibid.

20. J. H. Cassedy, "Muckraking and Medicine: Samuel Hopkins Adams," *American Quarterly* 16, no. 1 (1964): 85–99.

21. R. G. Hillman, "A Scientific Study of Mystery: The Role of the Medical and Popular Press in the Nancy-Salpetriere Controversy," *Bulletin of the History of Medicine* 39 (1965): 163–82.

22. M. Schudson, *Discovering the News*.

23. Ibid.

24. Ibid.

25. Ibid.

26. Ibid.

27. W. J. Kovarik, "The Ethyl Controversy: The News Media and the Public Health Debate over Leaded Gasoline, 1924–1926" (doctoral diss., University of Maryland–College Park, 1993–1994), abstract in *Dissertation Abstracts International*, 55 (04): 9425070.

28. Fine, *A Giant of the Press*.

29. Ibid.

30. Ibid.

31. Burkett, *News Reporting*.

32. Schudson, *Discovering the News*; and Berger, *Story of the New York Times*.

33. Ibid.

34. Ibid.

35. Hoehling, *The Great Epidemic*.

36. Burkett, *News Reporting*.

37. Berger, *Story of the New York Times*.

38. Ibid.
39. Ibid., and Fine, *A Giant*.
40. Fine, *A Giant*.
41. S. Baran and D. Davis, *Mass Communication Theory: Foundations Ferment and Future* (Belmont, CA: Wadsworth Publishing Co., 1995).
42. Ibid.
43. Berger, *Story of the New York Times*.
44. Ibid., p. 161.
45. Ibid., p. 163.
46. A. Rosenfeld, "The Journalist's Role in Bioethics," *Journal of Medicine and Philosophy* 24, no. 2 (1999): 108–29.
47. See, for example, S. Dunwoody, "The Scientist as Source," in *Scientists and Journalists: Reporting Science as News*, ed. S. M. Friedman, S. Dunwoody, and C. L. Rogers (New York: Free Press, 1986): 3–16; S. Dunwoody and M. Ryan, "Academic and Professional Training Patterns of Science Writers," *Journalism Quarterly* 52, no. 2, (1975): 239–90; S. Dunwoody and M. Ryan, "Public Information Persons as Mediators Between Scientists and Journalists," *Journalism Quarterly* 60, no. 4 (1983): 647–56; S. Dunwoody and M. Ryan, "Scientific Barriers to the Popularization of Science in the Mass Media," *Journal of Communication* 35, no. 1 (1985): 26–42; S. Dunwoody and M. Ryan, "The Credible Scientific Source," *Journalism Quarterly* 64, no. 1 (1987): 21–27; S. Dunwoody and B. T. Scott, "Scientists as Mass Media Sources," *Journalism Quarterly* 59, no. 1 (1982): 52–59; D. Nelkin, "An Uneasy Relationship: The Tensions Between Medicine and the Media," *Lancet* 347, no. 9015 (1996): 1600–1603; S. Ramsey, "A Benchmark Study of Elaboration and Sourcing in Science Stories for Eight American Newspapers," *Journalism Quarterly* 76, no. 1 (1999): 87–98; C. Russell, "The View From the National Beat," in *Scientists and Journalists: Reporting Science as News*, ed. S. M. Friedman, S. Dunwoody, and C. L. Rogers (1986): 81–94; J. Stacey, "The Press Embargo: Friend or Foe?" *JAMA* 254, no. 14 (1985): 1965–66; P. H. Tannenbaum, "Communication of Science Information," *Science* 140 (1963): 579–83; J. A. Winsten, "Science and the Media: The Boundaries of Truth," *Health Affairs* (Spring 1985): 5–23; and J. A. Winsten, "Promoting Designated Drivers: The Harvard Alcohol Project," *American Journal of Preventative Medicine* 10 suppl. 3 (1994): 11–14.
48. Burkett, *News Reporting*.
49. Ibid.
50. Burkett, *News Reporting*; and Winsten, "*Science and the Media*," 5.
51. Hoehling, *Great Epidemic*; and, Patterson, *Pandemic Influenza*.
52. M. Alvarez and R. Begue, "Eradication of Infectious Diseases"; V. Fulginiti, *The Millennium in Infectious Diseases: Focus on the Last Century 1900–2000*, http://www.medscape.com/Medscape/GeneralMedicine/journal/2000/v02.n02/mgm0331.fulg/mgm0331.fulg-01; B. G. Rosenkrantz "Cart Before Horse: Theory, Practice, and Professional Image in American Public Health, 1870–1920," *Journal of the History of Medicine* 29 (1974): 55–73; and P. Starr, *The Social Transformation of American Medicine* (New York: Basic Books, 1982).
53. Hoehling, *The Great Epidemic*.
54. Ibid.
55. Ibid., p. 22.
56. McNeill, *Plagues*.

57. Ibid.

58. See J. D. Brown and K. Walsh-Childers, "Effects of Media on Personal and Public Health," in *Media Effects: Advances in Theory and Research*, ed. J. Bryant and D. Zillmann (Hillsdale: Lawrence Erlbaum Associates, 1994): 389–416; R. J. Davis, "Epidemiology on the Agenda: The Framing of Chronic Health Risks by the News Media" (doctoral diss., Brandeis University, 1993), abstract in *Dissertation Abstracts International*, 54 (02): 9316011. Kovarik, *The Ethyl Controversy*; M. McCombs, "News Influence; T. Radford, "Influence and Power of the Media," *Lancet* 347 (1996): 1533–35; Rice and Atkin, "Principles of Successful Public Communication Campaigns"; D. Rubin and V. Hendy, "Swine Influenza and the News Media," *Annals of Internal Medicine* 87 (1977): 769–74; and P. Saliou, "Crises Communication in the Event of a Flu Pandemic," *European Journal of Epidemiology* 10, no. 4 (1996): 514–17.

59. See Beveridge, *Influenza: The Last Great Plague*; Davila, "La Gripe Española"; Hume, "The 'Forgotten' 1918 Influenza Epidemic" Hoehling, *The Great Epidemic*; and Kolata, *Flu*.

60. Alfred W. Crosby, *America's Forgotten Pandemic: The Influenza of 1918*. (New York: Cambridge University Press, 1989).

61. Kolata, p. 8.

62. Kolata, *Flu*.

63. Hume, *The Forgotten*.

64. Spratt, "Science, Journalism and the Construction of News: How Print Media Framed the 1918 Influenza Pandemic," paper presented at the annual meeting of AEJMC, Miami Beach, Florida, 7 August 2002.

65. Rubin and Hendy, "Swine Influenza and the News Media"; Saliou, "Crises Communication in the Event of a Flu Pandemic."

66. Krieghbaum, "Public Interest in Science News."

67. Schramm, *Science and the Public Mind*.

68. Tannenbaum, "Communication.

69. Ibid.

70. W. F. Miser, "Critical Appraisal of the Literature," *Journal of American Board of Family Practice* 12, no. 4 (1999): 315–333.

71. Ibid.

72. See G. A. Gellert, K. V. Higgins, R. M. Lowery, and R. M. Maxwell, "A National Survey of Public Health Officers' Interactions with the Media," *JAMA* 271, no. 16 (1994): 1285–89; E. F. Jones, J. R. Beniger, and C. F. Westoff, "Pill and IUD Discontinuation in the United States, 1970–1975: The Influence of the Media," *Family Planning Perspectives* 12, no. 6 (1980): 293–300; C. C. Mann, "Press Coverage: Leaving out the Big Picture," *Science* 269 (1995): 166; Satcher, "Prescription"; and D. L. Shaw and P. V. Van Nevel, "The Informative Value of Medical Science News," *Journalism Quarterly* 44, no. 3 (1967): 548.

73. G. Basky, "Media Coverage of Health Stories Often Inaccurate, MDs Report," *Canadian Medical Association Journal* 161, no. 4 (1999): 361; and D. Crouteau, "Examining the 'Liberal Media' Claim: Journalists' View on Politics, Economic and Social Policy (Including Health Care), and Media Coverage," *International Journal of Health Services* 29, no. 3 (1999): 627–55.

74. See P. H. Abelson, "Scientific Communication," *Science* 209 (1980): 60–62; D. P. Fan, "Impact of the Mass Media on Calls to the CDC National AIDS Hotline," *Inter-*

national Journal of Bio-Medical Computing 41 (1996): 207–16; S. Klaidman, *Health in the Headlines: The Stories Behind the Stories* (New York: Oxford University Press, 1991); Krieghbaum, *Public Interest*; D. S. Lane, A. P. Polednak, and M. A. Burg, "The Impact of Media Coverage of Nancy Reagan's Experience on Breast Cancer Screening," *American Journal of Public Health* 79, no. 11 (1989): 1551–52; N. Maccoby and J. W. Farquhar, "Communication for Health: Unselling Heart Disease," *Journal of Communication* 25, no. 3 (1975): 114–26; A. J. Sofalvi, "Mass Media and the Inglefinger Rule: Implications for Health Education," *Wellness Perspectives* 10, no. 1 (1993): 69–73; Tannenbaum, *Communication*; and Winsten, *"Promoting Designated Drivers."*

75. See J. S. Bowman and K. Hanaford, "Mass Media and the Environment Since Earth Day," *Journalism Quarterly* 54, no. 1 (1977): 160–65; B. J. Cole, "Trends in Science and Conflict Coverage in Four Metropolitan Newspapers," *Journalism Quarterly* 52, no. 3 (1975): 465–71; Davis, "Epidemiology"; V. S. Freimuth, R. H. Greenberg, J. DeWitt, and R. M. Romano, "Covering Cancer: Newspapers and the Public Interest," *Journal of Communication* 34, no. 1 (1984): 62–73; C. J. Glynn and A. R. Tims, "Sensationalism in Science Issues: A Case Study," *Journalism Quarterly* 59, no. 1 (1982); D. P. Phillips, E. J. Kanter, B. Bednarczyk, and P. L. Tastad, "Importance of the Lay Press in the Transmission of Medical Knowledge to the Scientific Community," *New England Journal of Medicine* 325, no. 16 (1991): 1180–83; W. R. Oates, "Social and Ethical Content in Science Coverage by Newsmagazines," *Journalism Quarterly* 50, no. 4 (1973): 680–84; J. T. Rich, "A Measure of Comprehensiveness in Newsmagazines Science Coverage," *Journalism Quarterly* 58, no. 2 (1981): 248–53; and R. G. Shepherd, "Science News of Controversy: The Case of Marijuana, *Communication Monographs* 62 (1979): 1–36.

76. See Davis, *The Ethyl Controversy*; and E. Singer, and P. M. Endreny, "Reporting on Risk: How the Mass Media Portray Accidents, Diseases, Disaster and Other Health Hazards," *Risk: Issues in Health & Safety* 4, http://www.fplc.edu/medindx.htm (2001); M. T. Maldonado, and M. Belsey, "Culture, Health and the Media," World Health (March/April 1996): 28–29; J. W. Schneider and P. Conrad, *Having Epilepsy: The Experience and Control of Illness* (Philadelphia: Temple University Press, 1983); S. Sontag, *Illness as Metaphor* (New York: Farrar, Straus and Giroux, 1978); S. Sontag, *AIDS and its Metaphor* (New York: Farrar, Straus and Giroux, 1989); and D. E. McGee, "Emerging Meanings: Science, the Media, and Infectious Diseases," *JAMA* 276, no. 13 (1996): 1095–97; R. Gregory, "Risk Perceptions as Substance and Symbol," in *Risky Business: Communication Issues of Science, Risk, and Public Policy*, ed. L. Wilkins and P. Patterson (New York: Greenwood Press, 1991): 1–10.

77. Singer and Endreny, "Reporting on Risk: How the Mass Media Portray Accidents, Diseases, Disaster and Other Hazards," *Risk* 15 (Summer 2001), http://www.fplc.edu/risk/vol15/summer/singer.htm; and D. Nelkin, "Forward: Why Is Science Writing So Uncritical of Science?" in *Risky Business: Communication Issues of Science, Risk, and Public Policy*, ed. L. Wilkins and P. Patterson (New York: Greenwood Press, 1999): xi.

78. S. Friedman, S. Dunwoody, and C. L. Rogers, eds., *Communicating Uncertainty: Media Coverage of New and Controversial Science* (Mahwah, NJ: Erlbaum Associates, 1999); Klaidman, *Health in the Headlines*; L. Wilkins and P. Patterson, eds., *Risky Business: Communicating Issues of Science, Risk, and Public Policy* (New York:

Greenwood Press, 1991); M. Moore, ed., *Health Risks and the Press: Perspectives on Media Coverage of Risk Assessment and Health* (Washington, D.C.: Media Institute, 1989); and Gregory, "Risk Perceptions," 1.

79. D. Nelkin, *Selling Science* (New York: W. H. Freeman, 1987).

80. M. Angell, *Science on Trial: The Clash of Medical Evidence and the Law in the Breast Implant Case* (New York: W. W. Norton & Co., 1996), 155.

81. Nelkin, "Forward," 53.

82. S. Priest, "Cloning: A Study in News Production, *Public Understanding of Science* 10 (2001): 59–69.

83. See S. E. Bird and R. W. Dardenne, "Myth, Chronicle, and Story: Exploring the Narrative Qualities of News," in *Media, Myths, and Narratives: Television and the Press*, ed. J. W. Carey (Newbury Park: Sage Press, 1988): 67–86; Davis, *Ethyl Controversy*, 1993; E. Goffman, *Frame Analysis: An Essay on the Organization of Experience* (Boston: Northeastern Press, 1986); Hume, "*The 'Forgotten'*", 77; and Pan and Kosicki, "*Framing Analysis*."

84. Bird and Dardenne, "Myth, Chronicle, and Story."

85. For the Spanish flu pandemic, January 1, 1917, through September 30, 1918, there were 47 articles. During October 1, 1918, through March 31, 1919, there were 219 articles. From April 1, 1919, through December 31, 1920, there were 152 articles. For the Asian flu pandemic, January 1, 1956, through September 30, 1957, there were 138 articles. During October 1, 1957, through March 31, 1958, there were 108 articles. From April 1, 1958, through December 31, 1959, there were 37 articles. For the Hong Kong flu pandemic, January 1, 1967, through September 30, 1968, there were 43 articles. During October 1, 1968, through March 31, 1969, there were 72 articles. From April 1, 1969, through December 31, 1970, there were 19 articles. Previous studies were not as comprehensive and tended to include only those stories from October through December.

86. McCombs, "*News Influence*," 1–16.

87. R. A. Logan, "Popularization versus Secularization: Media Coverage of Health," in *Risky Business: Communicating Issues of Science, Risk, and Public Policy*, ed. L. Wilkins and P. Patterson (New York: Greenwood Press, 1991), 43–59.

88. J. W. Chesebro, "The Media Reality: Epistemological Functions of Media in Cultural Systems," *Critical Studies in Mass Communication* 1, no. 2 (1984): 111–30.

89. Chesebro, "Media Reality."

90. K. Mannheim, *Ideology and Utopia: An Introduction to the Sociology of Knowledge* (New York: Harcourt, Brace and Co., 1936).

91. Mannheim, *Ideology and Utopia*, 10.

92. A. Schultz, "On Multiple Realities," *Philosophy and Phenomenological Research* 5 (1945): 551.

93. Berger and Luckmann, *Social Construction*.

94. Goffman, *Frame*, 1986.

95. Chesebro, "Media Reality,", 115.

96. Tuchman, *Malcing News*, and "Professionalism."

97. Priest, "*Cloning*"; and Pan and Kosicki, "*Framing Analysis*."

98. S. Horning, L. Walters, and J. Templin, "Voices in the News: Newspaper Coverage of Hurricane Hugo and the Loma Prieta Earthquake," *Newspaper Re-*

search Journal 12, no. 3 (1991): 32–45; Hume *"The 'Forgotten'"*; and Pan and Kosicki, *"Framing Analysis"*.

99. Bird and Dardenne, "Myth, Chronicle, and Story," esp. 67.

100. S. Kozloff, "Narrative Theory and Television," in *Channels of Discourse, Reassembled: Television and Contemporary Criticism*, ed. R. C. Allen (Chapel Hill: University of North Carolina Press, 1978), 67–100; S. Dunwoody, "Community Structure and Media Risk Coverage," *Risk* 15 (Summer 2001), http://www.fplc.edu/risk/vol15/summer/dunwoody.htm.

101. Angell, *Science on Trial.*

102. R. J. Davis, "Epidemiology on the Agenda: The Framing of Chronic Health Risks by the News Media," (Ph.D. diss., Brandeis University, 1993): 73.

103. Davis, "Epidemiology"; R. S. Sumpter and M. A. Braddock, "Source Use In A 'News Disaster' Account: A Content Analysis of Voter News Service Stories," *Journalism & Mass Communication Quarterly* 79, no. 3 (Autumn 2002): 539–58; Horning, Walters, and Templin, "Voices in the News"; D. Nelkin, "Journalism and Science: The Creative Tension," in *Health Risks and the Press: Perspectives on Media Coverage of Risk Assessment and Health*, ed. M. Moore (Washington, D.C.: Media Institute, 1989): 53–71.

104. Dunwoody, "Community Structure," Pan and Kosicki, "Framing Analysis"; Nelkin, "Journalism and Science."

105. Davis, "Epidemiology," 76.

106. Nelkin, "Forward," xi.

107. Bird and Dardenne, "Myth," 69.

108. Ziporyn, *Disease in the Popular American Press*, 5.

109. Angell, *Science on Trial*, 155.

110. W. G. Kirkwood and D. Brown, "Public Communication About the Causes of Disease: The Rhetoric of Responsibility," *Journal of Communication* 45, no. 1 (1995): 55–76.

111. Davis, "Epidemiology."

112. Nelkin, "Forward," ix–xiii.

113. Klaidman, *Health in the Headlines*, 5.

114. Nelkin, "Journalism and Science," 54.

115. Davis, "Epidemiology," 77.

ONE

INTRODUCTION

As early as 1799, Congress passed a quarantine act in response to several yellow fever outbreaks across the United States. During the mid-nineteenth century, cholera spread globally, with three outbreaks. In 1842, a British scientist discovered a link between environmental conditions and public health. During the 1840s, Britain passed several public health acts in order to improve the water supply. By the late nineteenth century, many diseases, such as diphtheria, tetanus, cholera, and tuberculosis, had been identified, and public health officials were beginning to formulate new approaches to public health prevention. In 1906, "Typhoid Mary," the most famous typhoid carrier, was discovered. In 1907, U.S. immigration officers began to routinely check newly arrived immigrants. If they were found to be sick, officers had the option to send them back.

In 1912, the United States set up its first public health services department. A year later, the U.S. Supreme Court ruled that the rights of individuals would be denied when an imminent health threat to the American public was perceived. Therefore, by the time the first great flu pandemic hit the United States in 1918, public health officers were armed with new medical knowledge and a legal right to take whatever measures necessary to contain and control any perceived public health threats.

EARLY COVERAGE

The *Readers' Guide to Periodical Literature*, the *New York Times Index*, and *Palmer's Guide to the London Times* first identified and indexed coverage of influenza for the years 1917 through 1920.[1] Although the *Readers' Guide to Periodical Literature* did have two articles about influenza listed under the year 1916 in its index for 1915 to 1918, it was not until the summer of 1918 that coverage of the emerging pandemic began and continued.[2]

Collier's, a weekly mass-produced magazine, ran an article in March 1916 by a physician who referred to influenza as "grippe."[3] The article detailed information about influenza symptoms and its prognosis. It was extremely interesting to note that in reference to an influenza epidemic, the article said:

> [T]there have been in the past great pandemics of grippe, since the sixteenth century . . . with a very considerable mortality and a grievous aftermath of chronic malaise and suffering.[4]

The article predicted influenza outbreaks would last "six to eight weeks during the winter," and said:

> Such mortality, such morbid sequelae, are not likely, however, to attend the 1916 epidemic because with successive experiences of any infection, its virulence and destructiveness are likely to be progressively modified.[5]

The article explained that one does not build a true immunity or tolerance to influenza and must take measures to avoid getting sick. The article noted that influenza is "highly contagious," and that public buildings or meeting places should be avoided during the height of the epidemic.[6] The article even mentioned public health policies in the last sentence, and said: "Spitting ordinances should be enforced, dust laid, ventilation established, and overcrowding of street cars prohibited."[7] This coverage, two years before the 1918 pandemic, clearly demonstrates that public knowledge, or frames about influenza epidemics, was clearly established. The mention of ordinances against spitting implies that this type of ordinance was in place before the 1918 pandemic.

BEFORE THE PANDEMIC: JANUARY 1917 THROUGH SEPTEMBER 1918

The first breaking story about influenza indexed for the *defined* time period for this study was in *The Times* (London) on April 12, 1917.[8] It was one sentence from the twelfth paragraph in a column about general news tidbits, titled "News in Brief," and said, "Deaths from influenza numbered 16, having been 41, 17, and 25 in the preceding three weeks, the average being 27."[9] From this we can see that the term influenza is a familiar one since it is not qualified and is included with information about another common deadly disease for the time period, measles. There are no more indexed stories in *The Times* referencing influenza for another year and three months. From this, one can assume that deaths from influenza were a common occurrence, as they were in

America. Hence, a mediated narrative existed well before the first pandemic.

Fourteen months after the London mention of influenza, in June of 1918, coverage about influenza began to appear in the *New York Times*. The coverage began with a report about a disease outbreak in China that resembled influenza, whose "sickness is not fatal, and it runs its course in four days."[10] Again, familiarity with the term influenza is established with U.S. coverage since the term influenza is also not further qualified.[11] The next *New York Times* article's summary blurb, taken from a cable from "the Hague," dated June 20, 1918, read, "Spain Affected by German Sickness and Other Countries Will Be, Says Hollander."[12] This was the first link to Spain for what would later become known as the Spanish Influenza. It is interesting to note that in the midst of World War I the disease was presented as a German sickness. Even though a source attribution is contained in the summary blurb, the person who predicted other countries would be affected by the German sickness is not mentioned anywhere in the body of the article. Several quotes contained in the article are from a "Dutch tailor who recently returned from Germany."[13] The Dutch tailor attributes the German sickness to a lack of nourishment, stating that the water accumulation on the sick person's body is "due to the enormous quantity of turnips now eaten by the Germans of all classes."[14] This type of narrative suggests that this mysterious disease was brought about by the Germans and aggravated by the typical German diet.

The next article in the *New York Times* made the front page and is reported within the context of World War I with a byline from a war correspondent.[15] It is not until the third paragraph that there is mention of influenza. The correspondent made use of the first-person narrative and said, "Their health does not seem of the best just now, and they are said to be suffering to some extent from a kind of influenza, to which they are perhaps rendered more liable by their restricted rations," and "This sickness is not, in my opinion, accountable for the delay in launching a new offensive."[16] Again, one can assume that there was a familiarity with the term influenza, with a focus on the Germans' sickness.

Two days later another front-page article mentioning influenza appeared within the same context.[17] However, now the flu is referred to as "Spanish Influenza," and believed that "it will be difficult to prevent further spread of the epidemic":[18]

> The disease prevalent in the German Army is reported to be of the new Spanish type, which recently broke out in Berlin and other German cities, and is presumed to have been brought to the trenches by men returning from leave.[19]

However, there is no mention of fatalities, only that the illness is spreading and might be due "to the shortage of German doctors and the conditions of under nutrition among the city populations."[20] The last paragraph was set off in parentheses and said that the prevalence of influenza was reported by Philip Gibbs in the *New York Times* two days before.[21] It is interesting to note that the editors felt that this article was of great news value and wanted to make sure that readers knew that the *New York Times* had already reported on this topic.

The next article was an opinion piece, with no byline, titled "Concerning Spanish Influenza," and appeared the following day.[22] The author's medical knowledge is evidenced by the lead sentence:

> What degree of importance should be ascribed to the report that an epidemic of "Spanish influenza" is sweeping through the German armies on the western front depends on the degree of virulence marking the particular strain of bacilli that is now at work.[23]

The article debated the merit of whether it would be deemed humane to hope that the flu took on a severe form, thereby eliminating the enemy and putting a quick end to the war. The author switched to a prophesying theme and said, "If the influenza is raging on one side on No Man's Land, it is sure to appear on our side of the lines."[24] The author returned to the idea that perhaps allies will not be affected if this flu strain is actually influenced by undernourishment.[25] The author then speculated about the name "Spanish" for this flu:

> The fact that this influenza is called Spanish by no means proves it of that origin. Dubious, too, is the recently suggested theory that the malady in its present form was started by the conditions produced among men making long cruises in submarines. Yet that theory may be true.[26]

In the same newspaper an opinion piece placed several sections before contained the headline, "No Influenza In Our Army."[27] The article simply reports that there are no cases of influenza among American troops stationed in Germany, that thousands could be affected at once, this might delay the war, and that "Precautions have already been ordered, however, to meet any emergency."[28]

As coverage picked up in New York, three months after the first story in *The Times* (London), on July 2, 1918, articles about influenza began to appear on a daily basis in London.[29] The July 2 article emphasized that Londoners were dying from a recent influenza attack, and great numbers of people were becoming suddenly ill, but they generally recovered after a couple of days of bed rest. Dr. R. C. Jewsbury, a Lambeth pathologist, was quoted in the article and said, "The prevalent Spanish influenza was very rapid at the onset, acute in its progress, and rapid in disappearing."[30] The pathologist recommended, as a preventative to influenza, that one take "about a teaspoonful of cinnamon oil and quinine every day."[31]

The article in the next day's issue was grimmer: "So far as numbers are concerned the present is the worst epidemic in the city (Manchester) for many years."[32] However, despite the report of deaths and increasing spread of the disease, the article balanced any fear by saying, "Happily, the recovery is quick under careful treatment" and "the Medical Officer of Health said the disease was, for the most part, of a mild character."[33] Therefore, at the onset of the influenza pandemic in London, the disease narrative produced a theme which expressed that while the disease may cause deaths, one would be okay if it was dealt with appropriately.

By July 6, 1918, *The Times* reported that "the influenza epidemic shows no signs of abating"[34] and on almost a daily basis during July, *The Times* reported fatalities in Great Britain.[35] War coverage by *The Times* during this time period also included several articles about Spanish influenza in Germany, India, and the Swiss army.[36]

On July 15, 1918, *The Times* ran a letter to the editor containing a request for *The Times* to rerun another letter to the editor by the same person from February 28, 1895, about influenza.[37] The letter addressed how one might ward off "la grippe." This "letter" actually establishes two previous frames: one, that influenza had been previously linked to Spain because the Spanish term for influenza is la grippe; and two, that influenza, at least during this particular man's lifetime, was experienced previously as a very hard-hitting epidemic during 1895. Therefore, influenza had a previous epidemic history in London; younger readers were now aware of it, and it had been previously associated as a Spanish disease.

The coverage about influenza stopped as suddenly as it appeared and did not resurface in *The Times* until September 12, 1918. Up until the beginning of the actual influenza season—October through March—the coverage was sporadic and consisted primarily of death statistics and the "reappearance of Spanish influenza" in Spain, Sweden, and India.[38]

Coverage about influenza began to appear in the *New York Times* with regularity during July 1918 and continued through December 28, 1920, with only one article in the last month of 1920.[39] It wasn't until September 1918, a month before the beginning of the "defined" time frame for the pandemic, that coverage also began to appear with some regularity in magazines indexed by the *Readers' Guide*. However, in cross-referencing the *Cumulative Subject Index to the Public Affairs Information Service Bulletins 1915–1974* (PAIS), government printed bulletins about the 1918 pandemic did not begin to appear until 1919, several months after the height of the

Spanish influenza pandemic in the United States. The medical bulletins were mainly reactionary in nature and usually reported statistics about the aftermath of the pandemic, different state health boards' reactions to the pandemic, and ways to prevent future pandemics.[40]

The coverage in the *New York Times* prior to October 1, 1918, focused primarily on how the epidemic was affecting the Germans.[41] One article blamed the epidemic on exhaustion, rather than a virus, and said the illness "which has been described as Spanish influenza, is really an illness due to hunger and consequent exhaustion."[42] On July 27, 1918, the reports began to detail the spread of the epidemic to the Swiss army.[43] It wasn't until August 14, 1918, that actual speculation about the spread of the influenza epidemic to the United States appeared as front-page coverage and developed into a mediated public health debate involving public health policy.[44] This story ran on the first page in the second column and contained details of a Norwegian ship that had landed at the New York City Port with ten sick passengers and reported that four passengers had died en route.[45]

The *New York Times* narrative presented a debate about how the New York Port authorities had let the ship pass quarantine, despite fatalities and ill passengers having been transported to a New York hospital. The debate continued two days later with reports about the involvement of New York City Health Board Commissioner Dr. Royal S. Copeland.[46] The next day, an editorial questioned the merits of conflicting information being reported by the health commissioner, the ship's doctor, and the attending physician for the sick passengers:[47]

> There may be doubts as to the protection accorded by our most efficient Quarantine Station and vigilant city health authorities, if after so many thousands of cases of Spanish influenza in Spain, in Germany, in France, in England, in Cuba . . . perhaps the health authorities of the port and the city have been a little too eager to reassure the public, which prefers the truth to official demulcents. And, possibly, those authorities have been too easy or incredulous in regard to our Spanish visitor.[48]

After the editorial, another article appeared with medical authorities defending their actions for the initial story that was run the day before.[49] The lead emphasized the frustration of the *New York Times* reporter, who said, "Eleven more cases of Spanish influenza, or whatever it is, were reported at Quarantine yesterday."[50] The article presented more conflicting information from health authorities about the Norwegian ship's sick passengers and that the port authorities would not call for a quarantine of ships with suspected cases of Spanish influenza because, as Dr. Leland E. Cofer, the health officer for the port, said:

> Spanish influenza is a misnomer. We have had epidemics of influenza in this country, with symptoms very like those of the cases developed in Spain. Yet the world didn't rise up and call it American or United States influenza. Nobody knows definitely whether this European variety that we have heard of recently is Spanish or Norwegian or Swedish or what.[51]

The information contained in this article is indicative of the frames that existed before the pandemic and the narrative created during this pandemic. First, it is obvious that influenza epidemics were not new to Americans. Second, at this time, the name of the disease, Spanish influenza, among health authorities is not an agreed upon term, and the origin of the disease has yet to be determined. Therefore, health authorities were not equipped with complete knowledge or medical expertise about the emerging pandemic. Later in the article, Cofer goes on to explain that America had bigger things to worry about than this outbreak:

> This country is at war and, besides having our hands in winning of the war, we have also the job of supplying our Allies with much that they need with which to enable them to fight on successfully. This port cannot be clogged for any minute longer than necessity requires. Therefore, when we find what may be called minor communicable diseases on ships entering the port, such as the ones I have spoken of, and to which must be added influenza, we simply report them to the city Board of Health. . . . There is not the slightest danger of an influenza epidemic breaking out in New York, and this port will not be quarantined against disease.[52]

In an article immediately following this article, titled, "Special to The New York Times," is a report dated for the previous day from Washington, D.C., that said the United States Public Health Service is aware of the reported cases of Spanish influenza in New York City, and that they "will take no steps to establish a quarantine against disease."[53] Therefore, the initial arbiters of Spanish influenza both by health authorities from New York City and the U.S. government, maintained that this form of influenza was not considered a threat and that they would not interfere with the business at hand, which was the world war.

The next day, August 17, 1918, an article in the *New York Times* said New York Health Commissioner Copeland was "ordering" Director L. I. Harris, of the Bureau of Preventable Disease, "to inaugurate, at once, a campaign against influenza and all such communicable diseases."[54] Here, is a clear case of a shift of responsibility from the New York City health commissioner to the U.S. public health director. Before the actual onset of influenza, the responsibility for dealing with the disease changed from a local problem to a U.S. government, or federal, problem. Additionally, the article said that ships would be responsible for identifying and reporting influenza cases to the local Board of Health, which would in turn track all infected immigrants and, whenever necessary, put the infected individual in isolation.[55] All physicians in New York City were requested to cooperate with the health department, and the "Sanitary Squad" was to renew its fight against public spitters. "Members of the Sanitary Squad received strict orders yesterday to arrest all offenders."[56] Despite the fact that port authorities had refused to quarantine infected ships, the New York Board of Health, through the direction of Dr. Copeland, had taken control of the situation. The article is framed as if New York City has just gone to war with the Spanish influenza. The shift from the previous day's coverage demonstrates a change in framing from *there's nothing to worry about* to *we have everything under control.* Regardless of the situation, the coverage served to alleviate the public from any worry or concern in reference to Spanish influenza. The next day, August 18, 1918, another ship, the *New York Times* reported, had come into the New York City port with twenty-one new cases of Spanish influenza.[57] The response from officials reported in the article was:

> Colonel J. M. Kennedy, Medical Corps, U.S.A., Chief Surgeon at the New York port of embarkation, said yesterday that some persons seemed to have the notion that the city and Quarantine guardians of health had only recently taken an interest in the possibilities of an epidemic here of either foreign or domestic influenza. "Why," the Colonel said, "the present publicity given to incoming influenza is publicity given to an old story. Ships having influenza have been arriving at this port six weeks or two months ago. . . .
>
> "We can't stop this war on account of Spanish or any other kind of influenza. . . .
>
> "Influenza, and the kind that is coming here is just like ours or that of any other country, is not at all dangerous, except when pneumonia develops. Pneumonia develops in a comparatively few cases, and few of those cases have fatal results, except where the patient has become debilitated through lack of proper food. The less this whole subject is agitated the better it will be for New York and the whole country and for our army overseas."[58]

The thematic narrative for the Spanish influenza pandemic was now set in what appears to be a very volatile topic for the press and its arbiters. First, Kennedy let us know that influenza is a common occurrence, and this type of influenza had been in New York for at least two months, which would place the beginning of the pandemic's hold at the same time as that in the United Kingdom and Europe. Then Kennedy said that the war was more important than a common strain of influenza, and that the only people likely to die were those who weren't taking care of themselves, by not eating "proper food."[59] Here, influenza is solidly defined as a common ailment. The blame for a fatality from the disease is placed on the victim, and public health is better served for New York, the country, and U.S. Army by focusing on something else. Hence, a leading medical authority framed Spanish influenza in a way that signified that the disease was not new and not worth talking about. Therefore, within one month, the disease was framed as both a serious public health risk that required a national campaign and policing of "spitting" persons *and* as not a topic of concern, with arbiters positioned in high-ranking medical and government institutions.

Despite the call to stop reporting on influenza, between Kennedy's response on August 18, 1918, and the beginning of the official flu season, October 1, 1918, more than sixty stories appeared in the *New York Times*. On August 19, 1918, an article reported that the New York port authorities were "keeping a strict lookout on incoming steamships from Europe whose passengers or crews might have developed Spanish influenza," and "it would be impossible to quarantine every vessel."[60] More conflicting coverage about Spanish influenza as an ailment of the past and yet new is explained:

> Americans who have had both the Spanish variety and the old-fashioned "grippe" of years ago, declare that the newer form is more malignant and leaves the system much weaker, which is the cause of so many deaths from pneumonia.[61]

The author of this article implied that he or she had interviewed passengers from a recent ship by saying, "Some passengers from Finland said the epidemic had spread all through Russia as far north as Archangel and thence to Sweden, Finland, Norway, and Denmark."[62] On August 20, 1918, again, the *Times* reported another ship for which "experts" identified Spanish influenza in twenty-one passengers, but it was a "mild form" and "every possible danger of the disease spreading has been eliminated."[63] There was a break in coverage until September 5, 1918, when a French ship arrived at the New York port and reported two deaths at sea due to Spanish influenza.[64] This time, the article said, the ship was detained seven hours and sixteen patients were sent to the hospital for observation:[65]

> The Captain of the ship said there were a number of cases among the longshoremen and others along the waterfront at the French port whence the vessel sailed, but in his opinion the Spanish influenza was brought on board by the two Italian passengers. It developed into pneumonia, which caused their death.[66]

At this point, Spanish influenza was being blamed on yet another racial group, and not just passengers, but the crew, were infected. Eight days later, a week after the reported deaths, an institutional response was given to the media with the headline and subhead, "City is Not In Danger From Spanish Grip," "Health Commissioner Says Persons Here Have Not Been Infected."[67] The situation is framed by the health commissioner in a way that lets the public know that everything is under control and that laboratories of the Department of Health are investigating in order to prevent future cases and to treat current cases. He said, "At present no better advice can be given than to tell any one who actually contracts Spanish influenza to go to bed immediately and to remain quiet."[68] This was the first mention that there was a possibility that local citizens could indeed contract Spanish influenza.

The next day, medical authorities on a national level acknowledged the threat of influenza and managed to have the Associated Press run a complete bulletin issued by Surgeon General Blue, "in order to reach physicians of the country without a day's delay," and

> because the last pandemic of influenza occurred more than twenty-five years ago, physicians who have begun to practice medicine since 1892 have not had personal experience in handling a situation now spreading through a considerable part of the foreign world and already appearing to some extent in the United States.[69]

Now, the *New York Times* Spanish influenza coverage was framed in a very serious and urgent fashion. The article reported that the reasoning behind the Surgeon General's wanting the bulletin run in the national press was because of a "sharp outbreak" of influenza in several United States Army camps near Mobile, Philadelphia, Boston, New London, and New Orleans.[70] Not only was the disease now presented as an urgent public health concern, but it was reported to be spreading all over the United States *and* there was now fear of a resulting pandemic. The bulletin, which was placed in the middle of this very long article, contained general clinical, diagnostic, and treatment information for physicians. As for the American public, Surgeon General Blue stated:

> The present outbreak of influenza may be controlled to more or less some extent by the intelligent action on the part of the public.
>
> Persons so attacked should go to their homes at once, get into bed without delay, and immediately call a physician.
>
> Treatment under the direction of a physician is simple, but important.[71]

In reference to whether port authorities should practice quarantines, Blue stated, "There is no such thing as an effective quarantine in the case of pandemic influenza."[72]

Here, one can see that Spanish influenza coverage was framed as if it were the responsibility of the American public to act intelligently in order to not contract the disease, and a quarantine, which would be a government response to Spanish influenza, would be futile. Over the course of approximately two months, Spanish influenza moved from a frame of government responsibility and that there was nothing to worry about, to a frame of individual responsibility where government authorities could not take effective action. This type of ping-ponging of frames within the narrative for Spanish influenza continued during the entire pandemic. A week after the appearance of the bulletin in the *New York Times* by the Associated Press, the same bulletin was indexed in the *Readers' Guide* as the first magazine article for this time period.[73] The same day as the news coverage, September 14, 1918, an article about Spanish influenza ran in *Literary Digest*, with a synopsis of an article from the *Journal of the American Medical Association*, which said, "Before the so-called 'Spanish influenza' strikes us, and authorities agree that we shall not escape it, a few facts about what it is and what it does ought to be acceptable."[74]

In response to the erratic shifting of frames in reference to definition, blame and responsibility, and public health policies, the *New York Times* printed an editorial on September 18, 1918, which said:

> This country is about to undergo the serious inconveniences and not inconsiderable dangers that accompany and follow an epidemic of the so-called Spanish influenza. That this new variant of the "grippe" with which we have been only too familiar in other years really originated in Spain is a matter of some doubt . . . but whether the latest form of an old malady is Spanish or not is a question of no practical importance. We know when it came here and by what ships it arrived. We also know that the guardians of our ports at first told us that there was no danger of an epidemic here, and a little later admitted that there was not a danger, but a certainty of it, and that we should have to endure the consequent ills as best we could, as quarantine measures, to be effective, would have to be so stringent as to work an intolerable interference with the conduct of our war businesses on land and sea.
>
> That was a rather humiliating confession for the representatives of medical and sanitary science to make in these days.[75]

Even though the *New York Times* clearly presented the shifting of narrative frames played out in its newspaper to date, it added to the confusion by attempting to define the disease as German rather than Spanish.[76]

By the end of September, the coverage established that Spanish influenza was an epidemic spreading rapidly throughout the United States. However, paradoxically, while numbers rose in relation to the infected and fatalities, medical authorities maintained that the spread of influenza was "in control," or "well in hand."[77] An editorial on September 27 summed it up: "It is lamentably evident that the malady called Spanish influenza is fast assuming the pandemic form in this country, and lamentably evident, too, that it is a really serious affliction."[78]

The next day, the number of deaths in New York City after twenty-four hours equaled the previous total since July 1 at twenty-seven.[79] Therefore, well before October 1, the Spanish influenza pandemic was well situated in the United States, and as Americans dealt with the pandemic, coverage of the pandemic adjusted.

DURING THE PANDEMIC: OCTOBER 1918 TO MARCH 1919

The *New York Times* coverage for the month of October 1918 focused on what public health officials were doing, and reported daily death statistics across the United States from October 12 to mid-November. Once it was established that the Spanish influenza pandemic was present in the United States, a new debate played out in the media over defining the severity of the disease and the government's response, on all levels (city, state, and national), to the disease. For each report of increasing deaths and rates of infection, another article from a medical official or institution countered with headlines such as "Influenza is Halted, Health Reports Show" and "Influenza Impedes Ship Production." On October 4, 1918, headlines such as "Grip Now Sweeping Forty-three States," "New Gains In Grip Here," and "Boston Epidemic Wanes," appeared on the same page.[80] This type of good news/bad news continued until the deaths really did begin to decline.

Another frame that emerged early in the pandemic was the New York City health commissioner announcing that a potential vaccine might be made available to "prevent future infection of inoculated persons."[81] This presented the medical institution as having a cure, or magic bullet, to eradicate Spanish influenza. However, before a vaccine could be used, the flu spread rapidly and forced local governments to take "drastic actions" by closing schools, stores, and theaters. In Chicago, the *Times* reported, police were mobilized to take action:

> In an effort to eradicate influenza in this city, the Health Commissioner and the Chief of Police today issued orders to every member of the Police Department directing him to arrest not only violators of the spitting ordinances, but every person found coughing or sneezing without using a handkerchief.[82]

The response to influenza varied across the United States accordingly. For example, in reference to a story local in New York City, Health Commissioner Copeland was quoted as saying

> I don't want to be in the position of giving an interview that would appear antagonistic to what Surgeon General Blue has said. He is dealing with the

> nation. He finds a variety of conditions while we face only one here. For instance, in Oswego, with 23,000 persons, there was found 3,500 cases today. Now if we have one-sixth of the population here affected with Spanish influenza we would have 1,000,000 cases. We have had about 6,000 cases here, while Philadelphia has had 20,000 and Boston 100,000. One half of the 6,000 cases here are in 600 homes.
>
> It has been the position of the Department of Health from the first that no individual is in danger if he or she escapes the mouth or nasal secretion of some other person who has it. We believe it is proper to keep the theatres and churches open if we can eliminate the sneezers, coughers, and spitters.[83]

Another headline appeared two days later saying, "Experts Disagree On Epidemic Here." Health officials were now debating amongst themselves about influenza, which reinforced the earlier frame that health authorities did not know how to deal with Spanish influenza and that they were not in control.[84] This continued over to an editorial the same day, which said:

> It is evident that the Health Department hesitates to be strenuous, because, as Dr. Copeland says, "This community is not stricken with the epidemic." But it may be if only half measures are taken. A stitch in time saves nine. The closing of the schools is a debatable question. Dr. Copeland's reasons for keeping them open are not altogether convincing.[85]

A day later, in Lexington, the Kentucky Board of Health ordered "all public assemblages, even including funerals" to be halted.[86] As the flu ravaged throughout the United States, the disease narrative switched from a focus on the spread of infection, to one of how one could combat or "fight Spanish influenza."[87] The shift in responsibility for care was redirected to the individual, when Surgeon General Blue said:

> The public [had] to "learn something about the home care of patients ill with influenza," in order, he said, to reduce unnecessary calls on physicians, who have been greatly overworked.
>
> With reports today showing the epidemic to be spreading in many parts of the country, he found an acute shortage of doctors and nurses everywhere to meet the urgent needs of the patients who are seriously ill.
>
> "The present generation," said the Surgeon General, "has been spoiled by having had expert medical and nursing care readily available."[88]

He made this statement despite the fact that the first medical bulletin issued by the Surgeon General told Americans to go home and immediately call the doctor when they became ill.[89]

International coverage, when present in the *New York Times*, generally dealt with death statistics.[90] However, one story that received attention was that two French scientists claimed to have isolated the germ causing influenza, and then a magazine article in *Scientific American* explained that, according to European scientists, the clinical picture of the current pandemic was identical to "the last pandemic of 1889," and "the influenza bacillus may be evading capture on account of faulty method of inquiry."[91]

In response to international coverage of medical advancements regarding the flu, combating the flu pandemic with a vaccine emerged again with headlines that claimed: "Grip in the Y. M. C. A. Checked by Vaccine," and "Vaccine Cuts Army Influenza Deaths."[92] The health commissioner for Chicago then ordered a "general vaccination of Chicagoans with antitoxine, and advised all persons to salute their friends, but not to shake hands."[93] A lengthy article on October 20 referenced a high-ranking Russian doctor who had handled two previous epidemics:

> "Thanks to the public health officials of this country, you appear to be on the eve of the practical application of a vaccine for the destruction of the influenza bacillus," he said. "As for any suggestions from me, I think your health authorities are on the right track."[94]

This type of narrative suggests that there was a need to frame America as having equally sophisticated medical institutions, and it reemphasized that U.S. medical authorities were regaining control. One article reported:

> Scientific information regarding the influenza epidemic now daily accumulating in the State Department of Health and elsewhere is to be correlated and made available to health officials and the medical profession through the action of Governor Whitman (New York).[95]

On October 21, coverage took another turn, and began to document the decline in influenza cases across the United States.[96] As the death and infection statistics began to decline and public bans began to be lifted, another frame emerged that had not been present before: reported fighting between government and medical institutions. An October 24 *New York Times* story with the headline, "1,450 New Cases Recorded, Largest Number for a Single Day Since Epidemic Began," said:[97]

> As bad as the situation is, it is not as bad as the figures would indicate, Dr. Copeland pointed out. "It is true," he said, "that today we have the worst record we have had yet, but, I regret to say, certain physicians are responsible for this, because they have dumped in upon us reports of cases that should have been reported days ago."[98]

An October 26 article reported:

> Governor Edge was asked to remove Dr. Jacob C. Price as State Director of Health of New Jersey yesterday by Mayor Gillen of Newark. The Mayor, ignoring an order of the State Health Department, lifted a ban on all places of assembly, which was to remain in effect during the influenza epidemic.
>
> In his letter to the Governor, Mayor Gillen says he understands that Dr. Price took action without waiting for a meeting of the State Health Commissioners, and issued the order closing up business places throughout the state.[99]

The next day, another article reiterated Dr. Copeland's accusation that the influenza statistics were obscured due to reporting problems by physicians with a summary blurb that said, "Now Officially Decided That Norwegian Steamship Brought the Disease Here." Even influenza vaccines were called into question by Surgeon General Blue, who warned in another article:

> Use of vaccines in combating or treating Spanish influenza has not gone beyond the experimental stage. . . .
>
> "The health service urges the public to remember that there is as yet no specific cure for influenza and that many of the alleged cures and remedies now being recommended by neighbors, nostrum vendors, and others do more harm than good."[100]

By November 1918, news coverage in the *New York Times* about Spanish influenza focused on its decline and what was expected for the future. Daily coverage dropped off for newspapers, but increased for magazines.[101] The total number of news articles for the month of October was approximately equal to the amount for November 1918 through to the defined end of the pandemic in April 1919.

On November 1, *The Times* (London) continued to run "District Reports" chronicling deaths in and around London.[102] However, these reports were authored "By A Medical Correspondent" and not only noted the decline in influenza cases, but also began a narrative of preventative public health advice in reference to influenza.[103] On November 5, the theme shifted to one of guarded optimism:

> The decline in the "influenza" epidemic continues generally, and is evident the worst has been experienced. The situation, however, remains serious, and in some of the large industrial centers the disease seems to have gained ground within the last few days.[104]

This was the first hint that something might actually be amiss and that perhaps the flu wasn't going away. This type of coverage continued through the month of November, shedding no new information. Instead, when death numbers were down, stories turned to looking at the past calamity and criticized what could have been done. In an article by the medical correspondent, a debate ensued about whether an early warning system was in place. The medical correspondent wrote:

> [T]he idea that the epidemic could not have been foreseen is finally disposed of. It was foreseen, and that by a very important official body, which actually drew the attention of the health authorities to the danger. The claim that adequate steps to meet it were not made cannot, therefore, be disputed on the ground that no warning was given.[105]

Nonlocal coverage was sparse during November and December in *The Times* (London). Coverage still tended to emphasize the severity of influenza in foreign or nonlocal areas, or reported medical breakthroughs. In November, one article reported that a Spanish doctor had isolated the Spanish influenza "germ," while another article, by an "English Correspondent," described the influenza epidemic in Spain:

> The Spanish frontier was closed owing to the epidemic, which the Spaniards assert comes from France.
>
> The epidemic is a most serious affair, affecting the whole of Spain, and the death rate is truly awful. . . .
>
> Treatment are without number—vaccines, antiseptics, inhalations, and the rest. One is disinfected wherever one goes. At Madrid they squirted my boots, overcoat, and a bit of one bag with formalin. The music-halls and theatres advertise the fact that they disinfect twice daily. All the people are very frightened.[106]

British coverage reiterated previous frames, such as the blame for the epidemic originating elsewhere, and that the international form of influenza is immense and frightening as opposed to local effects. Headlines such as "India Scourged By Influenza; Millions of Deaths" and "New Zealand Paralysis" maintained that things were worse off elsewhere. The influenza coverage in London took on a frightening theme when, on November 7, 1918, a significant rise in influenza deaths was noted in *The Times* for London.[107] By December 3, 1918, the increase in deaths was being framed as a "new influenza wave" in Great Britain.[108]

Another frame that emerged during the "new wave" was that of creating readily available cures for ailing influenza patients, particularly, alcohol. Under the headline, "Spirits For Influenza Patients," an article said that

> with reference to the need of spirits for medicinal purposes during the influenza epidemic [a]rrangements have been made by which it is hoped to provide immediately extra supplies for medicinal purposes without infringing the regulations made by the Liquor Control Board.[109]

While there had been mention of liquor, specifically whiskey, as a possible cure for influenza, most of the comments were brief. This was the first article to give a headline and entire story devoted to framing liquor as a *medicinal* drink.

On December 18, *The Times* medical correspondent ran an article estimating that "nearly 6,000,000 persons have perished of influenza and pneumonia during the past 12 weeks" worldwide, with a call for public health measures to prevent future calamities.[110]

The same type of media framing of local stories was also present in the *New York Times* for the month of November 1918. The local coverage consisted of declining death statistics and, aftercare plans for victims of the grip involving the discussion of new public health policies.[111] Magazine articles indexed for November also followed along the same frames. In an article by the *North American Review*, criticism abounded in reference to an early warning system: "There can be no excuse nor even pretext of lack of warning of the deadly plague that scourges us. Its threatened invasion was heralded in advance."[112] Other articles questioned the course of the pandemic and detailed death and infection statistics.[113]

November 8, one day after London reported an increase in influenza deaths, the *New York Times* ran the headline, "Influenza Up In City," for a story that said there was an increase of 614 new cases.[114] But that was it; the rest of the coverage for November chronicled the lifting of bans across the United States and that the epidemic was a thing of the past.[115] Statistics abounded, and several lengthy articles discussed the course of the pandemic during August, September, and October. As far as the news coverage was concerned, the Spanish influenza pandemic was framed as another unfortunate epidemic that perhaps public health officials could learn from, even though deaths from influenza outnumbered those in World War I.[116] A *New York Times* international article identified another flu epidemic in China that affected more than 8 percent of the population.[117] Therefore, for all apparent appearances, Spanish influenza in the United States was being framed as a thing of the past. At the same time, during the latter two weeks of November, London was experiencing a new wave of influenza.

While New York was reviewing the perceived past influenza pandemic, nonlocal news coverage for the month of December 1918 in the *New York Times* began to chronicle a reframing of a resurgent pandemic in other parts of the United States and around the world. On December 12, 1918, Surgeon General Blue issued a bulletin in an article giving a "warning to the country that the influenza epidemic was by no means ended, and, that all possible precautions against the disease should be taken."[118] The rest of this article explained that new cases of influenza were being reported in California, Kentucky, Ohio, Missouri, Mississippi, Washington, West Virginia, South Carolina, Vermont, Massachusetts, and Pennsylvania.[119]

On December 13, 1918, conflicts over the new outbreaks, with public health officials as the arbiters, reemerged in the narrative.[120] First, New York City's Health Commissioner Copeland was quoted saying that he did not think New York City would need to prepare for the latest outbreak of influenza:

> "I have no anxiety as regards this city," he declared. "We had at least half a million cases during the epidemic just ended and, with our systems of transportation, crowded surface cars and overcrowded and poorly ventilated subways, it is probable that practically every susceptible person was exposed to the disease during some period of the epidemic. . . .
>
> "I think we may expect to have this incidence of the disease for some time to come, but I have no fear whatever that New York City will suffer another epidemic—certainly there is no evidence at present of any recurrence of the disease in epidemic form."[121]

Another article on the same page reported health officers in Chicago were split on the influenza scourge, and the American Public Health Association was unable to agree on preventative measures.[122] The coverage of public health policies was presented as ambiguous and uncertain, and relayed anxiety on behalf of medical institutions to readers.

The next day the *New York Times* editorial staff reemphasized the frame of anxiety in a very sarcastic editorial entitled "This Time Action Is Demanded."[123] It said:

> It is pleasant to read, coming from an official in a place as high and responsible as is the Health Commissioner of America's greatest city, that there need be felt here no fear of another influenza epidemic in the near future. The reading would be considerably more pleasant, however, if it were not so easy to recall that no longer ago than last Fall Dr. Copeland as confidently told us all that in a population well fed and strong as ours the influenza would have no choice to assume epidemic form, and that, even if we did have a few cases of it, they would be light. A few weeks later the whole country was struggling with pestilence that cost it something like 400,000 lives and seriously interfered with the conduct of its activities, including those of war.
>
> At present, therefore, what would be pleasantest reading of all would be announcements of preparations to prevent another affliction of this sort and a vigorous education of the public and medical profession in whatever means science provides for protecting us from another desolating plague like the one which has just "burnt itself out."[124]

While reports of influenza infection and fatalities increased, experts debated "whether influenza masks and the closing of churches and places of amusement are practical measures to combat the spread of influenza."[125]

By the end of December, Boston was recording up to 454 new cases of influenza a day.[126]

Nonlocal international coverage in the *New York Times* was framed in a very dramatic way. One article, which was picked up from *The Times* (London) and ran two days after the initial story, reemphasized the need for alarm:

> The *Times'* medical correspondent says that it seems reasonable to believe that throughout the world about 6,000,000 persons perished from influenza and pneumonia during the last three months.
>
> Thus the correspondent points out, influenza has proved itself five times deadlier than war, because in the same period, at its epidemic rate, influenza should have killed 100,000,000. Never since the Black Death has such a plague swept over the world, he says, adding that the need of a new survey of public health measures has never been more forcibly illustrated.[127]

Another headline read, "Tahiti Builds Pyres of Influenza Dead," and the article described the situation:

> Influenza has turned the Island of Tahiti into a charnel place. At the crest of Papeete burn great pyres, with the stark, sheet-covered bodies of many natives waiting to be thrown into the glowing ashes of those who have been consumed by the flames.[128]

For the latter half of the pandemic—January, February, and March of 1919—news coverage dropped off considerably. The number of magazine articles did increase, but were again consistently longer versions of previous newspaper coverage. They tended to focus on the history of influenza and preventative measures, and they always reflected frames already established by newspaper articles.[129]

While *The Times* (London) reported that influenza deaths were on the decline in London during January 1919, articles in the *New York Times* tended to frame the influenza story in the past, looking toward a future cure. They focused on lessons to be learned, historical pieces about disease, and debated preventative measures such as masks.[130] One article in *The Times* (London) introduced a new frame as a result of the influenza coverage, which was a call for more health coverage. Newspapers, he said, have had for a long time a City page dealing with matters financial. Why not a health page under a responsible editorship? He did not mean the publication of "answers to queries," but "well-considered accounts of recent advances in preventative medicine."[131] The story ran with a headline that read "Influenza Masks," and a subhead that read "Health Editors For Newspapers." This type of story contextually emphasized the link from actual influenza coverage to preventative health coverage.

There was more nonlocal coverage in *The Times* (London), and it continued the previous trends toward drama and devastation in foreign lands. In an article about Cape Town, *The Times* wrote:

> Relief parties were organized, and the military were called out to dig graves. Doctors and nurses worked till they dropped, and others, to keep themselves well, never went to their homes, but slept somewhere else with the door locked, as otherwise they could get no sleep.[132]

Berne was reported as having nearly one-sixth of its population affected by influenza, and in the capital of Iceland, with a population of about 8,000, "about 600 people had died" and many more were infected.[133] Influenza cases in Australia were "increasing in virulence," with a mortality rate of 10 percent for Victoria, with "coastal shipping . . . coming to a standstill."[134] Another story about Australia said, "Certain soldiers who broke quarantine from the transport Argyilshire (*sic*) are being hunted down and rounded up in the city and surrounding country."[135] The next day a continuation of the story explained:

> Great excitement was caused in Sydney at noon owing to 1,000 soldiers, who had been disembarked from the transport Argyleshire (*sic*) at North head last night, breaking quarantine. Without warning, the men donned gauze masks, lined up, and, led by men of the 1st Batt., 1st Division, forced an exit from the inner enclosure. . . .
>
> The men were orderly and good humoured, but complained of the sleeping and food conditions. The State Commandant intervened and finally brought the soldiers by ferry steamer to the city, interring them in the cricket ground.[136]

One of the first articles to frame influenza with the possibility of influenza-infected animals was by the *Times's* (London) Canadian correspondent, who reported:

> Woodmen engaged in the bush in Northern Ontario declare that moose are dying from Spanish influenza. One man discovered the bodies of two moose lying near each other, neither of which showed any sign of external injury, while another bushman encountered a bull moose hardly able to travel from exhaustion. Whether influenza or not, the bushmen are convinced that there is some plague among the moose in the Thunder Bay district.[137]

To this point, soldiers and animals had only been connected to influenza in reference to combat, scientific experiments, and vaccines. This new information suggested that influenza had shifted to a broader societal scientific concern.

During February 1919, infection rates and deaths picked up again. In between the reports of deaths in and around Great Britain, the British medical correspondent reemphasized the frames of preventative public and individual health measures, and scientific advancements in isolating the influenza "germ."[138] In the preventative framing of influenza, a recurrent cure was the use of alcohol. The medical correspondent said, "The good effects of wine continue to be emphasized and most agree in selecting port as the best of these. Alcohol should in no circumstances be withheld."

On February 22, 1919, in a letter to the editor, whiskey was ambitiously framed as the cure for influenza with a suggestion for a potential health policy:

> Sir,—As a doctor with a large working-class practice I know well the work our silent force—the police—have done for sick, wounded, or on-leave soldiers and their relatives, hence one hesitates to give them more, but none could do it so well or so effectively. I suggest brandy and whiskey—indeed all necessary stimulants—should be immediately placed at every police station throughout the land, and distributed under doctors, certificates to the sick at all reasonable hours—placed there by the Government out of bond, and retailed at reasonable prices. Profit is no object, only the saving of life; and the urgency of the epidemic demands it.[139]

Debates about health policies continued and projected, vis-à-vis the coverage, that a ministry of health would be formed. *The Times* (London) medical correspondent wrote:

> The public has now grasped the fact that this epidemic has defeated the combined efforts of the world to control it, and has seen that new methods are necessary if similar events are not to take place in the future. This is the one good thing in a very bad situation. A few years ago it was almost impossible to arouse public interest in health matters. To-day public interest is boundless. . . .
>
> We should like to believe that the new President of the Local Government Board (of health) is framing a policy on the matter, for sooner or later a policy will require to be framed. . . .
>
> Disease is preventable. The public means, quite seriously, that it shall be prevented.[140]

Therefore, the information in this article is quite *literally* a frame for public health policy as a result of the Spanish influenza pandemic.

News coverage during the last month of the defined time period for the pandemic focused on science and future public health policies.[141] Other articles discussed the financial effects of the influenza epidemic in Great

Britain.[142] Another story reported that there was an outbreak of influenza among sheep, advancing the idea of a connection between influenza and animals:

> [V]eterinary inspector for Westmoreland County Council and the Board of Agriculture, has diagnosed an illness among sheep in that neighborhood as corresponding with the influenza epidemic in human beings. . . .
>
> When first attacked the sheep become dull and listless, with a slight cough and a high temperature. Later the cough becomes worse and breathing more difficult, until the victim collapses from heart failure. Several flocks are affected, and already many deaths have occurred.[143]

Nonlocal stories in *The Times* (London) continued to frame influenza in the same way as local stories, with exception to the telling of the devastation in India, in which "deaths from influenza in India as a whole in 1918 are calculated at 5,000,000 for British India and 1,000,000 for Indian States."[144] A couple of days later, on March 13, the *Times's* correspondent reported:

> Influenza was responsible for six million deaths, equivalent to more than half the mortality attributable to plague in the 22 years during which plague has been epidemic in this country. . . .
>
> Major White declares that while he would be the last to deny that the Indian health organization is in urgent need of expansion and reform, it must be acknowledged that if India had possessed health and medical organizations as efficient as those of most progressive countries it would have been impossible to effect much in checking the ravages of the disease. . . .
>
> [I]t can be stated without exaggeration that from 50 to 80 per cent of the total population have recently suffered from influenza.[145]

This type of coverage of nonlocal influenza stories typifies the frames created to date.

Coverage by the *New York Times* for the last three months of the defined time period for the influenza pandemic switched from focusing on death statistics for entire communities to accounts of individual institutions or families suffering from influenza. One story reported:

> Sister St. Denis of the Brooklyn Home for Crippled, Blind, and Defective Children, at this place, and six of her young charges died yesterday as a result of the epidemic of influenza that is sweeping through the institution. There are 350 children in the home. At least 250 of them are ill with influenza.[146]

Another article reported:

> Within eight days four members of the family of John Twomey have died of influenza and two other members are seriously ill at their home, 438 East 188th Street, and are not expected to live. . . .

> Last Thursday the father, 58 years old, Treasurer of the Chaplain Duffy Club of the Church of Our Savior, 183d Street and Washington Avenue, died of influenza, although physicians say grief over the death of other members of his family hastened the end.
>
> Another son and a daughter have since been stricken and will be unable to attend the funeral of the father tomorrow.[147]

This type of frame had not been represented before. Prior to these stories, if there was mention of a particular individual infected with, or dying from influenza, it was of a well-known person, and the story was brief, usually no longer than one sentence. A magazine article reported on the heroic efforts of women at home fighting the influenza epidemic and used war rhetoric to frame the point:

> A war here in the United States, a war that reached into practically every community in the country and took a toll of American lives twice as great as that taken by the war overseas, has raged through the early winter months. In the fight against influenza, which is not yet finished, devoted women have served in the front ranks and many of them, uninspired by the interest and honor that helped the dough-boy to act the hero, have gone down to death, if not unwept, at least unsung.[148]

At the end of February, when ships began returning American soldiers, reports began to appear of army men dying at sea due to overcrowding.[149] While these articles were indexed as influenza stories, they were not about influenza. The story only recounted that some soldiers had at one time been infected with influenza, while the rest of the coverage detailed welcoming parties for the soldiers.

The few remaining stories for this time period were lengthy and either discussed future preventative measures, or successful steps in combating the disease, sustaining previous frames. One article even predicted another epidemic.[150] The nonlocal coverage in the *New York Times* briefly mentioned death statistics and infection rates around the rest of the world, with the same story that ran in *The Times* about Tahiti and the scientific advancements being made by foreign scientists.[151]

Perhaps the article most telling of the attention and framing that the Spanish influenza pandemic received was in a *Scientific American* article by Wade W. Oliver, who wrote:

> Universal attention has been attracted to this malady because of its apparent recent outbreak in epidemic and pandemic form, erroneously termed "Spanish influenza." Conclusion has been worse confounded by loose statements in both the "lay" and "medical" press that "Spanish influenza" is really bubonic plague, or what is commonly spoken of as "the black death." In the rapidity of its spread, in its high mortality, and in certain of its manifestations in the body, the disease has somewhat simulated, in certain respects, the pulmonary form of

> plague, that dread scourge of the tropics. But just as one, or even several swallows, do not make a summer, so do certain similarities fail to establish the identity of two distinct diseases.[152]

AFTER THE PANDEMIC: APRIL 1919 TO DECEMBER 1920

After the flu season, in April 1919, coverage about the Spanish influenza pandemic essentially ceased, and when referred to, it was framed as the great influenza epidemic of 1918, generally as a historic reference to the past. Influenza coverage did continue and consisted primarily of trying to predict the next influenza "wave."[153] The next wave of influenza reported was in Australia the same month, and was referred to as the "new Australian influenza epidemic" by *The Times* (London).[154] There were only four articles indexed that described the new influenza as a much milder form of the 1918 pandemic.[155] During the later part of April, a new milder form of influenza was reported in London. The influenza epidemic was treated by the new Ministry of Health and *Times'* medical correspondent very cautiously during its onset.[156] Several articles reran previously framed information about preventative measures and said the current epidemic was a "mild," "new wave" of influenza.[157] On October 27, 1919, the new Ministry of Health issued its first public health bulletin covered by *The Times*.[158] The article concluded:

> Whilst the possibility of a fresh outbreak of influenza cannot be excluded, the data available do not at present afford any indication of an immediate recrudescence of the disease epidemic form.[159]

The Times medical correspondent discussed a new feature in reference to this new milder form:

> One of the features of the present influenza wave is the marked depression, which it leaves behind it. Many persons who imagine they have had "only a cold" find afterwards that they cannot regain their wonted spirits and remain weak and breathless. There is more than a probability that these have had a mild attack of influenza. . . .
>
> [S]o far as possible cases which have been recognized should be isolated till clear of infection and people who feel "seedy" should consult a doctor without loss of time.[160]

This article demonstrates a frame of guarded behavior regarding advice given by certain individuals and is focused more on preventative measures than reactionary measures.

One nonlocal article reported that French doctors now knew the cause of influenza, similar to what the *New York Times* reported, and right below the brief story is a response from *The Times's* (London) medical correspondent that said:

> This work would seem to corroborate that of the British investigators, who reached the conclusion that a filter-passing organism and not the Pfeiffer bacillus is the cause of influenza. Their work was fully reported in *The Times* during the early months of this year.[161]

This type of framing implies that what the French doctors were reporting was not new, and that the British could take credit for this particular discovery.

In October 1919, another story recounted a British physician who published an article in *The Lancet* about predicting the next influenza epidemic by correlating bronchitis and pneumonia cases. Again, the article reinforces the frame that the British were savvy scientists, and instead of reacting to epidemics, one should be able to predict when the epidemic will occur. As a precautionary action, a week before the beginning of what was predicted to be a new epidemic, the Health Ministry ran an advisory in the medical correspondent's column detailing information that, the correspondent pointed out, was a revised edition of a document formerly issued. This reinforced the idea that precautionary measures to be taken up by the public had not changed since the 1918 pandemic.

For the year 1920, there were only thirteen articles indexed by *The Times* (London). The first article chronicled "influenza waves" and presented a new approach to the possible origin of the Spanish influenza pandemic:

> By far the most comprehensive account of the great influenza epidemic which has yet appeared was issued last night in a Supplement to the annual report of the Local Government Board for 1918–19.
>
> The writer, Dr. Carnwath, traces the origin of the plague and throws doubt on the title "Spanish influenza," which was originally given to it. Influenza was prevalent in epidemic form in China and Japan in March 1918. It was not reported from Spain till May 1918. Moreover, "during the last few years sporadic outbursts attracting more than casual attention have been occurring in America, and in the late winter and early spring of 1918 some of the United States military camps were severely attacked." At Camp Funston 11,029 out of a total strength of 29,000 men were attacked between March 4 and 29, 1918. A small epidemic in Chicago also occurred and culminated in the week ended April 6, 1918, when 24 deaths took place. It would seem, then, that the disease may have originated in China and come to America, and from there to Europe. Or it may have originated in America and gone both East and West.[162]

The narrative of this article actually focused on a logical origin for the Spanish influenza pandemic rather than a reactionary one of blame. This is the first article to make a connection to the waves of sickness and travel patterns of the American Army. Yet, there is no mention of British involvement, which indirectly keeps the blame on foreign entities.

British headlines in 1920 tell how influenza was essentially framed during this year. First, on January 27, 1920, a headline reads: "Influenza Epidemic Probable: Some Cautionary Hints."[163] The next day, "The Next Influenza Epidemic: Health Ministry and Prevention," and by February 5, 1920, "Influenza: No Epidemic Yet."[164] Several more stories ran during the year in February and March, with precautions, a couple of mentions of light outbreaks, but no actual epidemic.[165] By October 1920, the few headlines remaining said, "The Great Epidemic Unsolved" and "Influenza In Monmouth: An Unfulfilled Prophecy."[166]

The last article for 1920 in *The Times*, however, demonstrated that the theme of fear and anxiety created by earlier coverage had not been lost or abandoned:

> A period of high barometric pressure with cold was followed early this week by rain and warmth. Suddenly the cold returned—and everybody has begun to cough and feel a sense of constriction in the chest. A number of cases of influenza broke out.[167]

Therefore, while another influenza epidemic did not strike Great Britain, the frames that began with the coverage of the Spanish influenza pandemic did not end.

Influenza coverage in the United States, however, did experience a significant increase during the last year of the Spanish influenza time frame studied. For the remaining months of 1919, only thirty-eight articles were indexed under influenza for the *New York Times*. In April, right after the flu season, the *New York Times* ran a story about changes in public health policies for New York, directly attributing the changes to the "after effects" of influenza.[168] Several stories recounted the financial effects of influenza and revisited death statistics as they were made available, similar to previous coverage.

Nonlocal coverage in the *New York Times*, on the other hand, chronicled several new influenza epidemics in the Belgian Congo, India, and Buenos Aires over the next several months, with a severe epidemic reported closer to home, in Alaska.[169] On July 13, 1920, an article reported that 95 percent of the native-Indian population of Bristol Bay, Alaska, was "wiped out by an epidemic of influenza."[170] The Buenos Aires epidemic story actually referred to the epidemic as "Spanish influenza," whereas the other stories do not *name* the epidemic.[171] In August, a warning for another "visitation" of influenza for New York City appeared in the *New York Times* and said:

> Dr. Royal S. Copeland, Health Commissioner, issued a warning yesterday to prepare for a recurrence of influenza. The history of epidemic shows, he said, a recurrence in the succeeding year, and so Dr. Copeland looks for a return of influenza some time in early October. Because of this the Commissioner of Health warns all to guard their health carefully, and those who are weak he advises to build up their strength to meet a possible influenza attack.[172]

This article is completely different from the earlier responses by Dr. Copeland. Instead of placating the public or trying to avoid anxiety, the new frame is to prepare for the worst. Copeland even singles out high-risk persons and warns them to take precautions. The drastic change in the resulting narrative even prompted an editorial by the *New York Times*, which stated:

> As if our existing troubles were not sufficiently numerous and serious, we are now warned that with the coming of September there is likely to begin another epidemic of influenza. Memories of our last experience with that malady are still vivid in innumerable minds, and they are terrible enough to make this prophecy more than alarming. There is no need, however, to be panic-stricken, for the forecast is of a possibility, rather than a certainty, or even a probability.[173]

Now, the *New York Times* editorial response has also reversed itself as arbiter, with the editorial attempting to reduce anxiety, rather than criticize the health commissioner for not doing enough.

Twelve days after Copeland's warning, a response from a Cincinnati health officer is picked up from the Associated Press by the *New York Times*:

> Recurrence of the influenza epidemic this Fall is unlikely, said Health Officer William H. Peters of Cincinnati yesterday, taking issue with Dr. Royal S. Copeland, New York Health Commissioner. The State and nation has been "pretty well immunized by the disease last Fall and Winter," said Dr. Peters. Epidemics of such character, as a rule, do not strike twice in the same place, he said.
>
> "Of course there will be instances of influenza, the same as we have had every year," he continued.[174]

Copeland was presented as an unreliable source, somewhat belittled by the information presented by the "health officer" in this story.[175] However, eighteen days later, in the next indexed story, Surgeon General Blue substantiates Copeland's warning (beginning with the lead):

> "Will the 'flu' come back this year?"
> This is the question, being asked by thousands of scientists and millions of laymen throughout the world, is discussed by Surgeon General Blue of the Public Health Service in an official bulletin, in which it is said that the plague probably will reappear, but not in as severe a form as last Winter.[176]

The influenza narrative in the *New York Times*, therefore, took on a tone of warning. However, this time, in referring to or framing the definition of influenza, the reporter called the potential disease "the Plague," which signified more terror than the popular term "Spanish" influenza. The next day, an article ran with "suggestions for guarding against disease."[177] However, instead of the suggestions coming from the health commissioner, they were attributed to the New York Association for Improving the Condition of the Poor, and "all having the approval of the physicians of the organization."[178] This signaled yet another definitive change in arbiter for public health, for the moment, and marked the first time an association provided advice in this role as arbiter.

The second day after Blue's "warning," another editorial said

> That the city, and the whole country, for that matter, is again and soon to go through the terrible experience of an influenza epidemic may or may not be true. Among health authorities and medical experts it is considered a probability that the justly dreaded malady is about to make another attack on the world, and the more lugubrious of them say or hint that those who escaped the disease before will have it this time. They will admit, however, that the near return of the affliction is not a certainty.[179]

This editorial placed the debate and responsibility for influenza among "health authorities and medical experts" regarding whether influenza would return.[180]

On September 21, 1919 Copeland is reported as working with "noted bacteriologists" in trying to come up with a vaccine. Within a week, another article on September 28 reported that influenza had spread across the United States.[181] This time it was reported as a "mild type" of influenza, which was considered to have reached "the proportions of an epidemic in any State."[182] By October 9, Copeland was reported to say, "The influenza situation does not justify the slightest alarm, or hardly comment."[183] Now the framing of influenza in reference to an institutional response had returned to the previous framing of the Spanish influenza pandemic of 1918. Additionally, in November 1919 a story from Youngstown, Ohio, called an outbreak of influenza among workmen at a steel company "Spanish influenza," but only reported that six cases had been taken to the hospital.[184] By the end of 1919, local coverage of this second wave of influenza in the *New York Times* reflected the panicked themes during the first wave of Spanish influenza.

Nonlocal coverage in the *New York Times* for the later part of 1919 chronicled the same scientific discoveries that *The Times* (London) had. However, in reporting the French "discovery" at the Pasteur Institute, the *New York Times* only ran the information from Paris, and did not add any additional information to frame the story differently.[185] In keeping with the established trend to define influenza as more severe elsewhere, a report that, "Vaccine is being prepared in large quantities at St. Mary's Hospital and other bacteriological centres in London for distribution throughout the United Kingdom," was picked up by the Associated Press.[186]

Other headlines chronicled the severity of the epidemic elsewhere: "Grip Epidemic Spreads in Bolivia," "Influenza in Spain Again," and "Grip is Epidemic in Japan." While the United States prepared for what was being framed as a "mild" flu, the narrative reinforced the frame that the flu was deadly and rampant in the rest of the world. Regardless of the difference in framing between local and nonlocal news, Americans anxiously awaited local news of the perceived influenza epidemic. They did not have to wait long. Coverage in the *New York Times* for January and February 1920 surpassed the amount of coverage for all previous months except October 1918. The first article for 1920 was a nonlocal piece on January 9, which referred to an influenza epidemic "in its most dangerous form" in Buenos Aires.[187] Ten days later, an article told of another deadly epidemic in Poland:

> Hundreds of persons are dying daily in Warsaw. . . .
>
> Red Cross doctors who had experience with influenza epidemics in the United States and France say they are amazed at the almost instant infection upon exposure and the quick development of the disease. Death in many cases occurs within twenty-four hours. Women and young people appear to be particularly susceptible.
>
> There is almost a constant succession of funerals at Warsaw, many of them being held at night.[188]

This article clearly presented the epidemic outside of the United States as not only very infectious, but very deadly too. However, this epidemic wave was not given a name yet.

On January 16, a story about an outbreak of influenza in Chicago appeared in the *New York Times*.[189] The article described this particular outbreak as "Chicago's influenza," and said that preventative sanitary measures such as "downtown sweeping done at night" would be undertaken.[190]

In the last paragraph, the health commissioner for Chicago said that he did not think influenza in Chicago would amount to epidemic proportions. This type of narrative is identical to early coverage of the Spanish influenza pandemic, which framed responsibility for the disease within the realm of the public health institution, and while it reported several deaths and raised an alarm, a public health officer placated the potential for fear.

Coverage in the *New York Times* for the later half of January followed a similar narrative pattern established by earlier coverage during the 1918 pandemic. Initial stories of influenza by the health commissioner, however, were significantly different. This time, Copeland "predicted there would be a recurrence of the disease which swept the country more than a year ago, and which is moving eastward from Chicago," but that the "visitation would be less serious than last year's."[191] Instead of trying to placate the public into believing there was absolutely no danger, this time Copeland framed influenza as a threat, but not as a deadly one. Therefore, from the onset, Copeland defined this influenza not as the Spanish flu, but as one originating from Chicago.

Over the next several days, beginning January 17, 1920 coverage consisted primarily of contrasting stories about "Chicago's" influenza outbreak and New York's preventative public health measures to ready the community and the subsequent outbreak.[192] Most of these stories ran on the same page, side by side. At the same time that influenza in the United States was being framed as "Chicago's" and as a mild form, reports of influenza cases from Europe were being referred to as "Spanish" influenza.[193] Again, the narrative framing device to delineate foreign influenza or nonlocal influenza as a more severe problem elsewhere was used.

On January 22, the framing of preventative and then subsequent public health measures by Copeland was firmly established for the remainder of this influenza outbreak. Stories reported that local government authorities were obtaining whiskey for medicinal purposes, and obtaining additional nurses in anticipation of a widespread epidemic.[194] These "danger spots" made the front page of the *New York Times* in a long article detailing the two issues, and how Copeland was going to deal with them. It should be noted whiskey was a major issue because the United States was in a period of prohibition. This meant that while it was popular for doctors to recommend whiskey "for medicinal purposes," it was also illegal to purchase it.[195] This issue actually introduced new frames and brought about several public health policy debates and changes.

An editorial on the same day these issues were reported said:

> The Health Commissioner should be commended for his action in taking the menace of an epidemic seriously. He would not be doing his duty if he dis-

> missed the danger lightly. Happily the influenza of 1920 does not seem to be virulent. If the people of this city heed Dr. Copeland, all will be well, or as well as can be expected at this season of the year.[196]

This is one of the first editorials that does not oppose Copeland's actions or suggestions, but actually supports him. The next day, influenza coverage made page one again, with the subhead, "Health Chief Urges Druggists to Sell Whiskey for Use in Fighting Diseases."[197] The article reported that the death rate was lower than in 1917, which was the last "normal" year for reported deaths.

This implied that the current influenza outbreak was a lot less deadly than the Spanish influenza pandemic of 1918. However, in evaluating this article, it is likely that the higher news value was given because whiskey was being made available to the public, not because of the epidemic itself. In the middle of the article, with a small boldface centered sub-subhead, that read, "Asks Druggists to Sell Whiskey," a long story detailed new issues involved with adopting a new public health policy to distribute whiskey.[198] The amount of words and space given to this debate actually outnumbered the space given to reporting any medical complications, such as deaths, from the influenza outbreak. Several issues presented as obstacles for Copeland before whiskey could be distributed included the hesitance of druggists to distribute whiskey because they did not want to be associated as "liquor-runners," and that "there was no law," per the prohibition enforcement agent, "to prevent a druggist from charging as much for the liquor as he saw fit, as long as customers were willing to pay the prices charged."[199]

Toward the end of this story, Copeland is reported to approve of

> [t]he establishment by the Government of distributing stations where whiskey might be dispensed to fight influenza.

And:

> [I]t is understood that the officials have no discretion in the elimination of the various legal steps necessary to procure liquor for medicinal purposes, even in the most urgent cases.[200]

The next day a headline on page three, from Washington, read: "Offers 'Wet' Measure to Aid Influenza Fight," in which the article said that Representative Sabath wanted to "relax restrictions on whiskey obtained on physicians' prescriptions for ninety days on account of the influenza epidemic."[201] The same day, another editorial ran discussing the "growing menace of influenza":

> In the shadow of another visitation druggists should put behind them their fear of being "identified with the liquor traffic." If time is lacking to convert them to a common sense view of the situation, the Federal Government should come forward with a plan to provide the whiskey legitimately at stations under its control. That is the proposal of Dr. Royal S. Copeland, the health Commissioner, and he should continue to urge it until relief is furnished.[202]

Influenza was now a means to overcome prohibition and to ride out the influenza epidemic "stimulated," so as not to become seriously ill.[203] However, given the nature of hindsight, was this perspective obvious then? One should consider that the rest of the coverage about the second influenza epidemic presented is that the epidemic is mild. Deaths were nowhere near those of the last pandemic, and, given coverage the year before that said that influenza was an annual expected visitor, one logically deduces that influenza created a frame to overcome the limitations of prohibition.[204] The whiskey issue was greatly enhanced by several page-one news stories with whiskey in the headline or subhead. On January 25, in the body of page-one story, there was a subhead that said, "Revenue Bureau Hastens Issuance of Licenses for Drug Stores to Sell Whiskey."[205] This is the first time the *New York Times* ran a banner headline on the topic of influenza. Furthermore, this is the first time that influenza had received this many page-one stories. Even in 1918, when thousands were dying weekly in New York City alone, there was no coverage that amounted to the type of coverage this outbreak received during January and February 1920. Therefore, while one cannot say there is a direct link, there most definitely is a relationship between the news coverage and resulting policy, because not only was a new public health policy initiated but a federal law was overridden, regarding alcohol.

The coverage through February continued to detail rates of infection across the United States, but there was a shift in the framing of the statistics, with actual deaths reported at the bottom of the story and rates of infection reported at the top of the story. The framing of this influenza epidemic, which did reach epidemic proportions, did not emphasize fatalities, but rather preventative measures being undertaken by public health officials, and that this influenza epidemic, while infectious, was not as deadly.[206] Dr. Copeland, as part of his preventative measures for public health, issued an appeal:

> To make it possible to obtain whisky in all sections of the city if influenza should become epidemic, the Internal Revenue Bureau took measures yesterday to facilitate the issuance of licenses to all reputable druggists.[207]

In the same article, after Copeland's "appeals," a debate ensued about whether to use vaccines:

> In an interview this morning Dr. Copeland seems to concede the efficacy of the pneumonia vaccine, both in the immunization and the treatment of pneumonia. A blind man ought to concede that now. But advice is given against the use of vaccines, because the influenza seems to be mild and produces no complications.[208]

Other health authorities disagreed with Dr. Copeland, and said it was too soon to label the current outbreak of influenza as "too mild" for a vaccine.[209]

Reports from other cities around the United States continued to frame the disease as "a mild type."[210] In the next page-one story, on January 26, Copeland used previous statistics from the 1918 epidemic and "predicted that the peak of the present outbreak would not be reached until the second week in February."[211] On the same day, two editorials were run in reference to influenza. The first said:

> In the matter of the influenza visitation, which already has become epidemic, the spread of the disease can be checked more by the thoughtfulness and precautions of individuals in the community than by measures of the Board of Health. Dr. Copeland is doing all in his power to protect the people of New York, but they must help themselves by co-operating with him.[212]

The editorial advised the public to stay away from crowded areas and curb their amusements while the epidemic was peaking. "But when the day's work is done, crowds can be avoided. It is not necessary to be more explicit," the editorial said.[213]

The second editorial spoke to Dr. Copeland's efforts to prevent a severe epidemic and called for the public to "scrupulously" follow all the rules published by the health commissioner.[214] The editorial staff was now solidly behind Dr. Copeland, which was not the case during the 1918 pandemic.

The next day, in another page-one story, the headline read: "Copeland Expects Rise in Influenza." The subhead said, "Monday Reports Show Only 1,712 Cases, but 3,000 Are Forecast Today," and the second subhead under it said, "New Working Hours Today—Spitters Warned—Virtues of Whiskey Discussed."[215] The information in the headlines implied that even though things might actually be better, they were not. Then, again, the "virtues" of whiskey are pronounced. Further down in the story, Dr. Copeland discussed the "controversy" that had "been made by newspapers outside the State and abroad regarding my attitude toward the use of whiskey in influenza."[216] He added, "it is not my business to advise treatment or criticize the methods of treatment of any disease; it is my business to prevent disease." By doing this, Copeland effectively removed himself from the responsibility of prescribing whiskey to patients, and left that "questionable burden" to practicing physicians. Therefore, while a public health institution was helping to facilitate the distribution of whiskey for "medicinal purposes," the narrative suggests that the institution was not the deciding or responsible party who issued the prescription—hence responsibility. Another article detailed the ordeal of filling a whiskey prescription:

> Speaking before the Medical Society of New York County in the Academy of Medicine, 17 West Forty-third Street, last evening Dr. L. W. Zwlsohn told of having difficulty in getting whiskey for patients.
>
> "We have the influenza epidemic with us and so is prohibition," he said. "I tried to get a prescription for whisky filled for a patient of mine. I tried a number of places and it was only after repeated efforts that I was able get as much as two ounces. For this my patient, who is a poor man, was charged $1.50. I move that we pass a resolution asking the Federal Government to suspend the regulations during the present epidemic so that the doctors can get whisky for their patients."[217]

While influenza continued to infect the population, the whiskey debate continued to be framed by the media as a problem to be overcome for influenza-afflicted persons. Headlines chronicled the plight for easy access to whiskey for influenza patients. On a page-one story January 28, one subhead read, "Prohibition Red Tape Cut for Druggists," and while many people were being infected by influenza, the cases continued as a "mild" type.[218]

The next day an article reported that the National Women's Christian Temperance Union "adopted a resolution condemning the use of whiskey in the treatment of influenza."[219] The article also included the opinion that aspirin was "very dangerous," too. This article, contextually, did not affect the whiskey debate. The article is on page 17, and placed next to an article about a man's claim to hear "messages from the dead."

A very long article ran on February 1 detailing the Volstead Act, which was a call for whiskey to be defined as a drug for medicinal purposes and in a way exempted from prohibition rules.[220] Under the subhead "A Way Around the Law," the article reported that the author of the bill was asked "whether any medical authorities had been asked for an opinion as to the framing of the medical part of the bill." His answer was no, because medical authorities are conflicted on this issue. The reporting here enhances the initial framing of whiskey and influenza. Many still were conflicted over the use of whiskey for medicinal purposes, but many still wanted an option other than prohibition. By the time the influenza epidemic ended, there was no other mention of whiskey or the Volstead Act in reference to stories indexed under influenza.

Page-one stories were still chronicling the daily infection statistics and fatalities for influenza and pneumonia cases up until February 1 in the *New York Times*. During February, articles reported a decline in influenza cases, and by February 5, that influenza was "on the wane."[221] During this time period, as stories began to report a decline in influenza in the United States, other nonlocal stories began to appear chronicling "new influenza forms" in Europe.[222] The subhead for one article exemplified the framing of nonlocal influenza: "Looks on More Serious Symptoms of Epidemic as Due to War Conditions." The article reported that "medical opinion here is inclined to the belief that the illness on this occasion will be more serious than formerly."[223]

As was the case with previous influenza coverage, as the rate of infection and deaths declined, so too did the news. Coverage changed back to a general discussion of statistics, financial concerns, scientific advances, historical overviews, and predictions for the next flu epidemic wave.[224] By February 15, Dr. Copeland announced that the 1920 influenza epidemic had been beaten, but would recur next year in a milder form.[225] The only editorial indexed for the remaining ten months was on July 29, and it tended along the narrative theme established by previous coverage outside of an epidemic time frame, which was to postulate on the past, note any new discoveries, and predict the future.[226]

On September 10, 1920, a *New York Times* article reported that the Public Health Service was on the lookout for a new epidemic, but that "there have been no indications of a return of last year's influenza epidemic this Winter."[227] The last article for the year, on December 28, reported on the possibility of an acquired immunity to subsequent epidemics or cases of influenza after having been through one epidemic.[228]

CONCLUSION

Narrative discourse for the Spanish influenza pandemic began with a definition in newsprint as a disease of concern for the Germans, and grew to be a public health fiasco for the United States and the rest of the world. The coverage clearly demonstrated that influenza was a disease that was well known internationally. It had a defined history and was, each year, anticipated by citizens and public health authorities. Several articles made reference to a pandemic that occurred between 1890 and 1895. However, as deaths began to mount during 1918, and a call for public health authorities to respond to the epidemic escalated, the disease went from a typical virus, to a "mystery disease" of insurmountable costs to lives worldwide.

The narrative discourse contained several different frames that placed blame for the actual disease, or influenza, virus from that of a "German sickness," to a health threat for impoverished people, to a health threat for all citizens.[229] Blame shifted from government institutions, to medical institutions, to individual lifestyles. By framing foreign or nonlocal influenza epidemics as being more severe elsewhere, this indirectly created blame for the foreign or nonlocal city. This was also another way to blame a racially different group. Nowhere, in any of the coverage for this pandemic, was there a mention of blame as a religious scourge or as a punishment from God. If anything, it was quite the opposite, in that influenza was framed to have been initiated by the Germans as germ warfare.

The coverage demonstrated that as the frame of influenza changed, so too did public health policies. For Great Britain, a Ministry of Health was created in response to the Spanish influenza pandemic in 1919. For New York, public health policy debates were aired in news stories and magazine coverage, and in editorials. Two significant shifts in public health policy were framed during the Spanish influenza pandemic: First, public health policies worldwide moved from reactionary ecological measures to medical and behavioral measures. Second, in the United States, as a result of influenza a federal law was challenged—prohibition.

However, as *The Times* (London) said, the public health philosophy to react to the disease, rather than anticipate it, helped to spur on medical research that focused on inoculation and vaccination. The problem was that the Spanish influenza virus had not been isolated and replicated in a suitable vaccine. This virus still presented a threat to public health, and as the last few news stories reported, still remained a mystery.

NOTES

1. See Appendixes A, B, and C for a detailed overview of the indexed material.
2. See the index under 1916.
3. J. B. Huber, "A Doctor's Point of View," *Collier's* (11 March 1916): 40.
4. Ibid.
5. Ibid.
6. Ibid.

7. Ibid.
8. The defined time period for this study is the complete years of 1917 to 1920 for the first pandemic. For further explanation, see chapter 3 of this study. "News In Brief," *The Times*, 12 April 1917, p. 3.
9. Ibid.
10. "Queer Epidemic Sweeps North China," *New York Times*, 1 June 1918, sec. 1, p. 3.
11. The fact that the word influenza is a recognized term for a type of illness is not really surprising, given the fact that the lexicon for "Spanish influenza" was established as early as 1647. See A. A. Hoehling, *The Great Epidemic* (Boston: Little, Brown and Co., 1961), prologue, for a more detailed explanation.
12. "Vienna Racked By Bread Riots; German Hunger Spreads Disease," *New York Times*, 21 June 1918, sec. 1, p. 7.
13. Ibid.
14. Ibid.
15. P. Gibbs, "Dysentery and Influenza Weaken German Army As Hopes of a West Front Victory Are Waning," *New York Times*, 25 June 1918, sec. 1, p. 1.
16. Ibid.
17. "Spanish Influenza Is Raging in the German Army; Grip and Typhus Also Prevalent among Soldiers," *New York Times*, 27 June 1918, sec. 1, p. 1.
18. Ibid.
19. Ibid.
20. Ibid.
21. Ibid
22. "Concerning Spanish Influenza," *New York Times*, 28 June 1918, sec. 10, p. 5. The article was probably written by one of the editors, since it is not identified as a "letter to the editor," as the surrounding pieces are. During this time period, it was a common practice for editorials to be placed on the same page as a letter to the editor with no byline.
23. Ibid.
24. Ibid.
25. Ibid.
26. Ibid.
27. "No Influenza in Our Army," *New York Times*, 28 June 1918, sec. 2, p. 1.
28. Ibid.
29. "Influenza Victims," *The Times* (London), 2 July 1918, p. 3. A page-three story is similar to a page-one story in the *New York Times*, in that page three of the London *Times* is the beginning of "news" coverage. The first two pages contained classifieds, including obits and then Parliamentary proceedings. Papers during World War I were not long and rarely contained advertisements. New York papers did not really change, except that additional sections were added for war coverage with elaborate illustrations. Illustrations during the war were rare in the London *Times*.
30. Ibid.
31. Ibid.
32. Ibid.
33. Ibid.

34. "Influenza Outbreak," *The Times*, 6 July 1918, p. 3.

35. "The Influenza," *The Times*, 9 July 1918, p. 3. "218 Death From Influenza," *The Times*, 11 July 1918, p. 3. "News in Brief," *The Times*, 15 July 1918, p. 3. "News in Brief," *The Times*, 16 July 1918, p. 3. "News in Brief," *The Times*, 17 July 1918, p. 3. "287 Deaths From Influenza in London," *The Times*, 18 July 1918, p. 6.

36. "Influenza Spreading in Germany," *The Times*, 4 July 1918, p. 5. "Influenza in Enemy Countries," *The Times*, 5 July 1918, p. 5. "Influenza in India," *The Times*, 8 July 1918, p. 7. "Influenza Among German Prisoners," *The Times*, 23 July 1918, p. 8. "11,500 Influenza Cases In Swiss Army," *The Times*, 24 July 1918, p. 5.

37. "Influenza," *The Times*, 15 July 1918, p. 9.

38. "News in Brief," *The Times*, 12 September 1918, p. 3. "News in Brief," *The Times*, 20 September 1918, p. 3. "Influenza and Dysentery," *The Times*, 18 September 1918, p. 8. "Spread of Influenza," *The Times*, 27 September 1918, p. 5. "1,000 Influenza Deaths," *The Times*, 28 September 1918, p. 5.

39. See appendix 1.

40. See R. Matteson Blackmore, ed., *Cumulative Subject Index to the Public Affairs Information Service Bulletins 1915–1975*. (Arlington: Carrollton Press, 1975): 534–35.

41. See "Germans With Fever Drop in Their Tracks," *New York Times*, 9 July 1918, p. 7. "Kaiser Ill of Influenza," *New York Times*, 11 July 1918, p. 2. "Rain Increases German Troubles," *New York Times*, 13 July 1918, p. 1. "Germans Die of Hunger," *New York Times*, 14 July 1918, p. 6. "All Meetings Forbidden During the Epidemic of Grippe," *New York Times*, 23 July 1918, p. 4. "Epidemics in Germany," *New York Times*, 26 July 1918, p. 20.

42. "Germans Die of Hunger," *New York Times*, 14 July 1918, p. 6.

43. "Spanish Grip on Swiss," *New York Times*, 27 July 1918, p. 13. "Red Cross to Aid Swiss," *New York Times*, 9 August 1918, p. 11.

44. "Spanish Influenza Here, Ship Men say," *New York Times*, 14 August 1918, p. 1.

45. Ibid.

46. "No Quarantine Here Against Influenza," *New York Times*, 15 August 1918, p. 16.

47. "Spanish Influenza," *New York Times*, 16 August 1918, p. 6.

48. Ibid.

49. "Health Head Calls Influenza Inquiry," *New York Times*, 16 August 1918, p. 16.

50. Ibid.

51. Ibid.

52. Ibid.

53. "Special to The New York Times," *New York Times*, 16 August 1918, p. 16.

54. "Orders Fight on Influenza," *New York Times*, 17 August 1918, p. 5.

55. Ibid.

56. Ibid.

57. "Liner Had 5 Deaths Due to Influenza," *New York Times*, 18 August 1918, p. 9.

58. Ibid.

59. Ibid.

60. "Epidemic Guard For Port," *New York Times*, 19 August 1918, p. 5.

61. Ibid.

62. Ibid.

63. "Spanish Influenza Found in 'Mild Form,'" *New York Times*, 20 August 1918, p. 20.

64. "Influenza Kills Two on Liner from Europe," *New York Times*, 5 September 1918, p. 22.

65. Ibid.

66. Ibid.

67. "City is Not in Danger from Spanish Grip," *New York Times*, 13 September 1918, p. 7.

68. Ibid.

69. "Takes Steps to Stop Influenza Spread," *New York Times*, 14 September 1918, p. 13.

70. Ibid.

71. Ibid.

72. Ibid.

73. "The Epidemic of Spanish Influenza," *Science* 48 (September 1918): 289.

74. "Spanish Influenza," *Lit. Digest* 58 (September 1918): 21–22.

75. "More Likely German Than Spanish," *New York Times*, 18 September 1918, p. 12.

76. Ibid.

77. "Influenza Epidemic Hits Camp Devens," *New York Times*, 15 September 1918, p. 14. "Spread of Influenza Checked in the City," *New York Times*, 23 September 1918, p. 9. "65 Deaths At Camp Devens: But Surgeons Believe Illness There is Under Control," *New York Times*, 24 September 1918, p. 9.

78. "A Danger Too Late Realized," *New York Times*, 27 September 1918, p. 12.

79. "New Cases in the City Doubled," *New York Times*, 28 September 1918, p. 10.

80. "Influenza is Halted, Health Reports Show," *New York Times*, 1 October 1918, p. 24; "Influenza Impedes Ship Production," *New York Times*, 3 October 1918, p. 24; "Grip Now Sweeping Forty-Three States," *New York Times*, 4 October 1918, p. 24; "New Gains in Grip Here," *New York Times*, 4 October 1918, p. 24; and "Boston Epidemic Wanes," *New York Times*, 4 October 1918, p. 24.

81. "Tells of Vaccine to Stop Influenza," *New York Times*, 2 October 1918, p. 10.

82. "Drastic Rule in Chicago," *New York Times*, 4 October 1918, p. 24.

83. "Conditions Different Here," *New York Times*, 5 October 1918, p. 6.

84. "Experts Disagree on Epidemic Here," *New York Times*, 7 October 1918, p. 7.

85. "The Spanish Influenza," *New York Times*, 7 October 1918, p. 12.

86. "Influenza Halts Grand Circuit," *New York Times*, 9 October 1918, p. 12.

87. See for example: "U.S. Bureau Seeks Cause of Influenza," *New York Times*, 11 October 1918, p. 11; "In fight on Influenza," *New York Times*, 11 October 1918, p. 11; "State Officials to Plan Fight on Epidemic Here Today," *New York Times*, 11 October 1918, p. 11; "Fight Stiffens Here Against Influenza," *New York Times*, 12 October 1918, p. 13; "How to Fight Spanish Influenza," *Lit. Digest* 59 (12 October 1918): 13–14; "Spanish Influenza and its Control," *Survey* 41 (12 October 1918): 45; "Copeland Names Committee to Act," *New York Times*, 13 October 1918, p. 18; "Federal Force Ready for Fight on Epidemic," *New York Times*, 15 October 1918, p. 10; "Copeland Asks Aid In Influenza Fight," *New York Times*, 16 October 1918,

p. 24; "Extent and Control of the Influenza Epidemic," *Survey* 41 (19 October 1918): 63–64; "Red Cross Active in Influenza Fight," *New York Times*, 20 October 1918, sec. 2, p. 2.

88. "Surgeon General Asks for More Home Care," *New York Times*, 13 October 1918, p. 18.

89. On September 14, 1919, Surgeon General Blue told Americans to call upon physicians as soon as they were sick. "Takes Steps to Stop Influenza Spread," *New York Times*, 14 September 1918, p. 13.

90. See "France Suspends Day Expresses," *New York Times*, 25 October 1918, p. 7; "Influenza in Copenhagen," *New York Times*, 25 October 1918, p. 7; and "Epidemic Grows in Argentina," *New York* Times, 26 October 1918, p. 11.

91. "Bacteriology of the Spanish Influenza," *Scientific American* 86 suppl. (October 1918): 249; "Say They Have Isolated Germ," *New York Times*, 15 October 1918, p. 10; and "Identify Influenza Germ," *New York Times*, 16 October 1918, p. 24.

92. See "Grip in the Y.M.C.A. Checked by Vaccine," *New York Times*, 17 October 1918, p. 9; and "Vaccine Cuts Army Influenza Deaths," *New York Times*, 18 October 1918, p. 24; "Vaccine a Success at Camp Dix," *New York Times*, 23 October 1918, p. 7; and "Big Firms Take up Fight on Influenza," *New York Times*, 23 October 1918, p. 8.

93. "Orders All Vaccinated," *New York Times*, 19 October 1918, p. 24

94. "Fought Influenza in Six Epidemics," *New York Times*, 20 October 1918, sec. 3, p. 5.

95. "To Study Influenza," *New York Times*, 23 October 1918, p. 8.

96. "Influenza Cases Drop 305 in City," *New York Times*, 21 October 1918, p. 12; "Influenza Shows a Decrease in City," *New York Times*, 22 October 1918, p. 9; "Cases Drop in Army Camps," *New York Times*, 22 October 1918, p. 9; "Draft Calls Resumed," New York Times, 23 October 1918, p. 5; "Epidemic Subsiding in Many Localities," *New York Times*, 25 October 1918, p. 22; "Vigilance Urged As Grip Wave Recedes," *New York Times*, 26 October 1918, p. 10.

97. "Delays In Reports Swell Grip Figures," *New York Times*, 24 October 1918, p. 12.

98. Ibid.

99. "Mortality Figures Explained," *New York Times*, 26 October 1918, p. 10.

100. "Beware of Sure Cures," *New York Times*, 27 October 1918, p. 14.

101. See appendix A.

102. "The Epidemic," *The Times*, 1 November 1918, p. 3.

103. See "The Epidemic," *The Times*, 1 November 1918, p. 3; "The Epidemic," *The Times*, 2 November 1918, p. 7; and "Epidemic Waning," *The Times*, 4 November 1918, p. 5.

104. "Influenza Mystery," *The Times*, 5 November 1918, p. 3.

105. "Epidemic Foretold," *The Times*, 6 November 1918, p. 3.

106. "Spain's Visitation," *The Times*, 8 November 1918, p.

107. "Rise in 'Influenza' Death-Roll," *The Times*, 7 November 1918, p. 3.

108. "New Influenza 'Wave,'" *The Times*, 3 December 1918, p. 3.

109. "Spirits For Influenza Patients," *The Times*, 10 December 1918, p. 5.

110. "6,000,000 Deaths," *The Times*, 18 December 1918, p. 5.

111. "Influenza Reaches Low Mark," *New York Times*, 1 November 1918, p. 24; "After Car Plans for Victims of Grip," *New York Times*, 2 November 1918, p. 11; and "Trade and Travel Back to Old Hours," *New York Times*, 3 November 1918, p. 6.

112. "Micawber: Sanitarian," *North American Review* 208 (November 1918): 657–60.

113. See "Spanish Influenza," *Scientific American* 119 (November 1918): 356; "Extent and Cost of Influenza," *Survey* 41 (November 1918): 63–64; "The Influenza Pneumonia Pandemic in the American Army Camps During September and October, 1918," *Science* 48 (November 1918): 451–56; and "Scientific Events," *Science* 48 (November 1918): 487–89.

114. "Influenza up in City," *New York Times*, 8 November 1918, p. 15.

115. "Cleveland Lifts Grip Ban," *New York Times*, 10 November 1918, p. 8; "Epidemic A Thing of Past," 14 November 1918, p. 12.

116. See the discussion in "Epidemic Lessons Against Next Time," *New York Times*, 17 November 1918, sec. 3, p. 10; and "Influenza Deaths Far Exceed War Losses," *New York Times*, 18 November 1918, p. 8.

117. "Influenza in China, Too," *New York Times*, 28 November 1918, p. 6.

118. "Influenza Reviving All Over The Country," *New York Times*, 12 December 1918, p. 13.

119. Ibid.

120. "Influenza Epidemic not Expected Here," *New York Times*, 13 December 1918, p. 9; and "Health Officers Split on Influenza Scourge, *New York Times*, 13 December 1918, p. 9.

121. "Influenza Epidemic not Expected Here," *New York Times*.

122. "Health Officers Split on Influenza Scourge," *New York Times*.

123. "This Time Action is Demanded," *New York Times*, 14 December 1918, p. 16.

124. Ibid.

125. "Experts to Study Influenza," *New York Times*, 14 December 1918, p. 10.

126. "Influenza at a High Mark," *New York Times*, 28 December 1918, p. 18.

127. "6,000,000 Died of Influenza," New York Times, 20 December 1918, p. 24.

128. "Tahiti Build Pyres of Influenza Dead, *New York Times*, 25 December 1918, p. 6.

129. See, for example, "How the 'Flu' Mask Traps the Germ," *Lit. Digest* 58 (December 1918): 21; "Expert Medical Advice on Influenza," *Lit. Digest* 59 (December 1918): 23; and "Vaccination Against Influenza," *Lit. Digest* 59 (December 1918): 25.

130. "Lesson of Influenza Epidemic," *The Times*, 2 January 1919, p. 3; "War Cures," *The Times*, 20 January 1919, p. 5; and "Influenza Masks," *The Times*, 30 January 1919, p. 5.

131. "Influenza Masks," *The Times*.

132. "Dying By Hundreds," *The Times*, 6 January 1919, p. 7.

133. "640,000 Influenza Cases," *The Times*, 18 January 1919, p. 7; and "Influenza in Iceland," *The Times*, 24 January 1919, p. 8.

134. "Influenza Ravages in Australia," *The Times*, 19 February 1919, p. 7.

135. "The Austrailasian Epidemic," *The Times*, 20 February 1919, p. 7.

136. "Army Influenza Riot," *The Times*, 21 February 1919, p. 9.

137. "Influenza Among the Moose," *The Times*, 27 January 1919, p. 7.

138. "The Smallest Germs," *The Times*, 7 February 1919, p. 5; "Lesson of 'After Effects,'" *The Times* 19 February 1919, p. 8; "Fighting the Epidemic, *The Times*, 20 February 1919, p. 5; and "The Prevention of Influenza," *The Times*, 22 February 1919, p. 10.

139. "Stimulants and Influenza," *The Times*, 22 February 1919, p. 10.

140. Influenza and Its Lessons: Clear Health Policy Needed," *The Times*, 25 February 1919, p. 7.

141. See "Influenza and Its Prevention, *The Times*, 1 March 1919, p. 7; "The Influenza Germ," *The Times*, 5 March 1919, p. 7; "The Influenza," *The Times*, 7 March 1919, p. 7; "Influenza Germ," *The Times*, 24 March 1919; and "The Problem of Influenza," *The Times*, 26 March 1919, p. 9.

142. "Effect of the Epidemic on Mortality," *The Times*, 7 March 1919, p. 7; "Influenza and Pauperism," *The Times*, 8 March 1919, p. 7.

143. "Influenza Among Sheep," *The Times*, 10 March 1919, p. 4.

144. "6,000,000 Deaths," *The Times*, 11 March 1919, p. 9.

145. "Influenza Worse Than Many Plagues," *The Times*, 13 March 1919, p. 9.

146. "Seven Die of Influenza," *New York Times*, 14 January 1919, p. 5.

147. "4 of Family Die in 8 Days," *New York Times*, 9 February 1919, p. 8.

148. "War-Reports from the Influenza Front," *Lit. Digest* 60 (February 1919): 62–67.

149. See "1,526 on Cruiser Here from France," *New York Times*, 21 January 1919, p. 6; "Storms Buffeted Troops on 4 Ships," *New York Times*, 23 February 1919, p. 5; "Influenza Attacks Troops on Voyage," *New York Times*, 6 March 1919, p. 6; America in with 4700 of the 27th," *New York Times*, 14 March 1919, p. 5; and "Influenza on Cruiser *Tacoma*," *New York Times*, 19 March 1919, p. 5.

150. "Influenza Chief Cause of Deaths in Home Camps," *New York Times*, 26 January 1919, sec. 3, p. 4; "Influenza Epidemic and Low Resistance," *New York Times*, 16 February 1919, sec. 3, p. 8; "Sing Sing Had No Deaths," *New York Times*, 23 February 1919, sec. 4, p. 11; and "Influenza Epidemic And Low Resistance," *New York Times*, 16 February 1919, sec. 3, p. 8.

151. "Egypt Ravaged by Influenza, *New York Times*, 5 January 1919, p. 3; "Stricken Tahiti," *New York Times*, 5 January 1919, sec. 3, p. 1; and "Influenza Virus Found," *New York Times*, 6 February 1919, p. 14.

152. "Influenza—The Sphinx of Diseases," *Scientific American* 120 (March 1, 1919): 200.

153. "Influenza 'Waves,'" *The Times*, 11 April 1919, p. 10.

154. "New Australian Influenza Epidemic," *The Times*, 3 April 1919, p. 11.

155. "An Influenza Vaccine," *The Times*, 4 April 1919, p. 11; "Sydney Again Masked," *The Times*, 7 April 1919, p. 11; and "Influenza," *The Times*, 8 April 1919, p. 11.

156. "Influenza and the Heart," *The Times*, 21 April 1919, p. 7.

157. "How To Keep Fit," *The Times*, 3 October 1919, p. 5; "A 'New Epidemic,'" *The Times*, 20 October 1919, p. 9; and "Mild Influenza Wave," *The Times*, 22 October 1919, p. 9.

158. "Slight Increase in Influenza," *The Times*, 27 October 1919, p. 9.

159. Ibid.

160. Ibid.

161. "Cause of Influenza," *The Times*, 21 October 1919, p. 11.

162. "Influenza Waves," *The Times*, 15 January 1920, p. 9.

163. "Influenza Epidemic Probable," *The Times*, 27 January 1920, p. 12.

164. "The Next Influenza Epidemic," *The Times*, 28 January 1920, p. 12; and "Influenza," *The Times*, 5 February 1920, p. 12.

165. "Influenza Warning," *The Times*, 27 February 1920, p. 9; and "Influenza Increasing," *The Times*, 25 March 1920, p. 13.

166. "Toll of Influenza," *The Times*, 8 July 1920, p. 11; and "Influenza in Monmouth," *The Times*, 5 October 1920, p. 7.

167. "Cold And Influenza," *The Times*, 3 December 1920, p. 9.

168. "Name Health Committee," *New York Times*, 6 April 1919, p. 11.

169. "Belgian Congo Swept by Influenza," *New York Times*, 25 April 1919, p. 10; "Influenza Sweeps India," *New York Times*, 26 April 1919 p. 3; "Grip Epidemic in Buenos Aires," *New York Times*, 5 July 1919, p. 7; and "Influenza Sweeps Alaska Natives," *New York Times*, 7 June 1919, p. 24.

170. "Plague Killed 95 Per Cent," *New York Times*, 13 July 1919, p. 3.

171. Ibid.

172. "Warns of Influenza," *New York Times*, 15 August 1919, p. 6.

173. "They May Again be Mistaken," *New York Times*, 16 August 1919, p. 6.

174. "At Issue with Copeland," *New York Times*, 27 August 1919, p. 9.

175. Ibid.

176. "Influenza Return Expected by Blue," *New York Times*, 14 September 1919, p. 4.

177. "Fresh Air Enemy of 'Flu,'" *New York Times*, 15 September 1919, p. 11.

178. Ibid.

179. "To Guard Against Influenza," *New York Times*, 16 September 1919, p. 14.

180. Ibid.

181. "Combine to Hunt Influenza Germ," *New York Times*, 21 September 1919, sec. 2, p. 13; and "300 Cases Reported," *New York Times*, 28 September 1919, p. 5.

182. "300 Flu Cases Reported," *New York Times*, 28 September 1919, p. 5.

183. "Few Influenza Cases," *New York Times*, 9 October 1919, p. 19.

184. "Influenza in Steel Mills," *New York Times*, 15 November 1919, p. 24.

185. "Finds Invisible Microbes Most Active in Influenza," *New York Times*, 20 October 1919, p. 17.

186. "British Prepare for Influenza," *New York Times*, 30 October 1919, p. 17.

187. "Influenza Sweeps Ship," *New York Times*, 9 January 1920, p. 34.

188. "Influenza Scourges Poland Striking Hundreds Dead Daily," *New York Times*, 19 January 1920, p. 15.

189. "Chicago Alarmed by Influenza Spread," *New York Times*, 16 January 1920, p. 12.

190. Ibid.

191. "Copeland Predicts Influenza Return," *New York Times*, 17 January 1920, p. 11.

192. See "523 New Cases in Chicago," *New York Times*, 17 January 1920, p. 11; "Chicago Influenza Epidemic Spreads," *New York Times*, 18 January 1920, p. 14; Ninety New Cases of Influenza in City," *New York Times*, 20 January 1920, p. 15;

"Influenza Shows a Large Increase," *New York Times*, 21 January 1920, p. 32; and "Influenza Cases Increase in Chicago," *New York Times*, 21 January 1920, p. 32.

193. "Influenza Cases on Liner," *New York Times*, 18 January 1920, p. 14; and "Ninety New Cases of Influenza in City," *New York Times*, 20 January 1920, p. 15.

194. "Influenza Cases Rise 462 in Day," *New York Times*, 22 January 1920, p. 1.

195. Ibid.

196. "The Return of the Influenza Menace," *New York Times*, 22 January 1920, p. 16.

197. "1,000 New Cases of Influenza Here," *New York Times*, 23 January 1920, p. 1.

198. Ibid.

199. Ibid.

200. Ibid.

201. "Offers 'Wet' Measure To Aid Influenza Fight," *New York Times*, 23 January 1920, p. 3.

202. "Need of Whisky for Influenza Cases," *New York Times*, 23 January 1920, p. 12.

203. "1,000 New Cases of Influenza Here," *New York Times*, 23 January 1920, p. 1

204. See previous coverage discussed for 1917 and 1918, and "Influenza Nears Epidemic Stage," *New York Times*, 24 January 1920, p. 1; "City's Business Hours Changed in Fight on Influenza," *New York Times*, 25 January 1920, p. 1.

205. "City's Business Hours Changed in Fight n Influenza," *New York Times*, 25 January 1920, p. 1.

206. "Influenza Cases Grow Throughout Country," *New York Times*, 25 January 1920, p. 2; "Mild Epidemic in Boston," *New York Times*, 27 January 1920, p. 3; "Influenza Gains 3,663 Cases in Day, with 57 Deaths," *New York Times*, 28 January 1920, p. 1; and "5,589 New Cases in One Day Break Influenza Record," *New York Times*, 29 January 1920, p. 1.

207. Ibid.

208. Ibid.

209. Ibid.

210. "Philadelphia, Washington, and Memphis," *New York Times*, 25 January 1920, p. 2.

211. "2,855 New Cases of Influenza; 30 Deaths Reported," *New York Times*, 26 January 1920, p.1.

212. "Checking the Influenza Spread," *New York Times*, 26 January 1920, p. 6.

213. Ibid.

214. "The Health Commissioner Shows the Way," *New York Times*, 26 January 1920, p. 6.

215. "Copeland Expects Rise in Influenza," *New York Times*, 27 January 1920, p. 1.

216. Ibid.

217. "Whiskey for Patients, *New York Times*, 27 January 1920, p. 3.

218. "Influenza Gains 3,663 Cases in Day, with 57 Deaths," *New York Times*, 28 January 1920, p. 1.

219. "Attacks Whiskey As Cure," *New York Times*, 29 January 1920, p. 17.

220. "Liquor As Medicine," *New York Times*, 1 February 1920, sec. 3, p. 10.

221. "Nurses' Pay Raised By Bids, Say Cooler," *New York Times*, 5 February 1920, p. 17.

222. "Europe Suffers From New Influenza Forms," *New York Times*, 1 February 1920, p. 7.

223. Ibid.

224. See "Ten Million Deaths in 'Flu' Plague a Year Ago," *New York Times*, 1 February 1920, sec. 9, p. 1; "Influenza Deaths Increase In City," *New York Times*, 4 February 1920, p. 19; "Influenza Deaths Fewer This Year," *New York Times*, 6 February 1920, p. 25; "Influenza Epidemic Passes the Peak," *New York Times*, 9 February 1920, p. 28; "Predicts Early End of Epidemic Here," *New York Times*, 10 February 1920, p. 32; and "Influenza Beaten, Says Dr. Copeland," *New York Times*, 15 February 1920, p. 14.

225. "Influenza Beaten, Says Dr. Copeland," *New York Times*, 15 February 1920, p. 14.

226. "Influenza Worst of Diseases," *New York Times*, 29 July 1920, p. 8.

227. "Influenza Danger Lighter," *New York Times*, 10 September 1920, p. 18.

228. "Public Health Service Reports Sufferers Free from Recurrence," *New York Times*, 28 December 1920.

229. "German Hunger Spreads Disease," *New York Times*, 21 June 1918, p. 1.

Two

INTRODUCTION

Between the Spanish influenza pandemic of 1918 and the beginning of the Asian flu pandemic of 1957, many changes took place in public health philosophies and practices. In 1928, when he first began studying influenza, British bacteriologist Sir Alexander Fleming discovered penicillin. In 1932, the electron microscope was invented, allowing viruses to be seen for the first time. In 1940, penicillin was finally isolated and manufactured into an antibiotic that has since revolutionized the way physicians treat bacterial infections. It proved particularly effective during World War II in the control of venereal diseases, which had been a major hindrance in previous wars.

The World Health Organization (WHO) was set up as an agency of the United Nations in Geneva in 1942 to help combat infectious diseases. In 1945, a vaccine was created and used effectively for influenza virus A and B. The World Health Organization initiated an influenza alert system in 1949. A successful polio vaccine was developed and put into use in 1953. When the Salk polio vaccine became available, long lines of people formed at the clinics that were administering the new vaccine, and in some cases riots ensued.

It was also during this period that the hydrogen bomb was being tested, plans were being made to put a man on the moon, and civil rights movements were taking hold. Cold War paranoia was at an all-time high with reports about Communist Russia and "Red" China at the forefront of daily news. The development of an antibiotic to fight bacterial infections and vaccines to prevent infections changed the way infectious diseases were combated. Vaccines and penicillin were seen as two scientific advancements that, like a magic bullet, could prevent or kill diseases that had previously plagued mankind. Therefore, optimism about anything scientific was de rigueur for this time period.

BEFORE THE PANDEMIC: JANUARY THROUGH DECEMBER 1956

The first indexed story related to the 1957 pandemic was a short historical piece in the magazine *Today's Health*, dated January 1956.[1] The article emphasized that a pandemic similar to that of 1918 was unlikely because of the development of an influenza vaccine and a worldwide "alerter system" whose purpose was "to get the jump on epidemics before they become pandemics" which started in 1949.[2] The article said that "thanks to modern drugs and vaccines, and an international alerter system," the great world tragedy of the influenza scourge of 1918–19 might never be repeated.[3] The article framed scientific advances as an optimistic approach to future public health threats, and set the thematic tone for the coverage to follow.

The first hint of a problematic outbreak of influenza was found in several stories by *The Times* (London) in 1956. On February 16, 1956, a *Times* correspondent said,

> Bristol is experiencing one of the worst influenza epidemics of recent years. . . .
> A spokesman for the British Medical Association said to-day: "Work is proving extremely heavy for us. In many cases whole households are infected. I cannot remember a worse attack in the city since 1941, and then we were understaffed."[4]

This first article introduced two frames to the narrative of influenza. First, a medical spokesperson was the arbiter, rather than a doctor or official. Second, the article let the reader know that there had been another bothersome influenza attack in 1941, eleven years prior to the 1957 pandemic. Therefore, it was apparent that influenza was still a threat to English communities, and a past reference established this frame.

During March of 1956, *The Times* (London) briefly mentioned two influenza epidemics in Geneva and Iceland.[5] On March 17, an article ran about a possible influenza epidemic at a boy's school in Dorset, Great Britain, but said, "There is no truth in rumours that the school will have to close down. The influenza does not appear to be of a serious type."[6] This article framed influenza at this point as posing no threat, since it was assumed that the virus was not serious. There are no other reports, so it appears that they were right.

In August of 1956, the *New York Times* ran its first story about a new vaccine reporting a 50 to 70 percent rate of effectiveness for warding off influenza.[7] This was the first framing of a weapon against the "war on grippe." It is interesting to note that the rhetoric of war was still being used in reference to influenza, as it was during World War I with the Spanish influenza pandemic. One explanation for this type of rhetoric could be that the vaccine was developed using U.S. Army men and recruits for the field trials in testing the vaccine. Another explanation could be that with the extensive amount of coverage that the Spanish influenza pandemic received during World War I, the war rhetoric of battling disease became an established frame over time, especially, when considering that previous news coverage about disease epidemics, pandemics, and plagues was closely associated with major battles and wars (since the Roman Empire).

The *New York Times* vaccine story was written by Bess Furman, who was one of the first bylined authors for a story about influenza.[8] Furman gave a detailed account of influenza viruses, and demonstrated that much had been learned about influenza since the 1918 pandemic. She said:

> When the development of the vaccine was originally announced, Health Service scientists said its purpose was to immunize against three types of grippe-producing A. P. C. viruses, so called because the symptoms are adenoidal, pharyngeal and conjunctival. Today's announcement referred to them as adenoviruses, "formerly designated as A. P. C. viruses."
>
> "The new designation of adenovirus was adopted for general use last May by the nation's leading investigators in the field of respiratory virus research," it explained. "The term replaces the several names that had been applied to the same group of viruses over the past few years."[9]

Nine months later, December 14, 1956, a news story ran in both the *New York Times* and *The Times* (London) about an epidemic of influenza in the Tokyo area, affecting more than 13,000 people, with 130 deaths.[10] These stories marked the beginning of the Asian influenza pandemic of 1957.

COVERAGE PRIOR TO THE PANDEMIC: JANUARY THROUGH SEPTEMBER 1957

A January article in *Changing Times* predicted that another wave of influenza was overdue and that a vaccine could be problematic, especially if the vaccine could not be produced before the epidemic hit.[11] This type of information raised awareness and was incredibly accurate in its predictions. However, once newspaper coverage began, all magazine articles essentially retold the news, or presented a reiteration of frames established by newspapers.

At first, the influenza epidemic in Hong Kong was treated like previous reports about influenza in newspapers: cautiously. One small story appeared in March, three months after the first story in Hong Kong, and said, "Polish medical authorities today ordered emergency measures to fight an influenza epidemic."[12] Another article appeared, almost a month later, and told of how Hong Kong was battling the "worst epidemic outbreak in years."[13] The article was framed within the context of current politics and showed how the effects of Communist China sentiment exacerbated the situation:

> The influx of an estimated total of 700,000 refugees from Communist China has created a constant danger because of over-crowded conditions. Fires and epidemics are the worst fears of the Government authorities.
>
> Throughout the day, thousands of sick persons have stood in long lines awaiting treatment in clinics. Many women carried glassy-eyed children tied to their backs.[14]

The article also reported that health authorities did not mandate reports to be made on virus infections, with numbers affected just estimates. This emphasized the frame that a foreign country was not as prepared to deal with an epidemic, as was the case with the United States, which had a mandatory reporting system.

Several weeks later, on May 2, 1957, it was reported that Taipei authorities feared the spread of influenza to Taipei and other Chinese Nationalist cities.[15] The article said that four hundred thousand cases of flu had already been reported in the port city of Keelung. These stories were the beginning of the *New York Time's* chronicling of the spread of influenza across the Asian continent.

By June, the epidemic had spread across China, Taiwan, Singapore, the Philippines, Indonesia, and India, and it had earned itself a name: the Far Eastern influenza virus.[16] On June 4, a U.S. public health service spokesman said, "Today there 'is a good chance' the epidemic influenza that has been sweeping the Far East, 'will be introduced into this country if it hasn't been.'"[17] Up to this point, the current influenza epidemic belonged to the Far East where it was described as having stricken nearly 20 percent of the populations it affected, closing schools and businesses along its path. The only description was that it was rapid and affected many, especially school-age children.

After Washington released a public service announcement of impending danger, an Associated Press wire story, originating from London, announced that the influenza epidemic currently "sweeping the Far East" was likely to spread to Britain and continental Europe.[18] With news that the epidemic was likely to spread, a new frame emerged, replacing a previous frame of death and destruction. Two days after it was reported that the influenza epidemic was likely to spread to the United States, an article said, "[W]hile a large number of persons have been stricken, deaths have been relatively few."[19] The new framing of influenza was, while it was very infectious with a sudden onset, it was not as deadly.[20] The next day, a longer article by Kennett Love, a correspondent from London, explained that Britain was speeding up research to develop a vaccine for the "new virus in Far East areas."[21] He said:

> A research doctor at the World Influenza Center here said serological tests at the center on samples flown here from Hong Kong showed that the virus was a hitherto unknown form.
>
> He described the new virus as fairly mild. Deaths have occurred mainly among young children and very old persons, but only a small fraction of cases have proved fatal so far, he said.
>
> The research scientist said the new strain definitely was much less dangerous than the influenza type that killed thousands throughout the world in three rapidly succeeding waves during World War I.[22]

This was the first comparison of the current epidemic to the previous pandemic of 1918. The framing of the article emphasized that, while the flu virus was new and not cloned for a vaccine yet, it was mild and not as deadly as the Spanish influenza virus. Love also pointed out the influenza's new name, Far Eastern influenza virus. Again, the framing of the disease placed the name and identity of the disease with a foreign country. Historically, the Far East and Red China were associated with American fears during the Cold War. As a result, one could assume that not only was Red China, or the Far East, a threat to democracy, but a health threat too. While this was not stated implicitly, it was implied with this type of framing device or rhetoric.

The day after, a headline in the *New York Times* said, "U.S. Acts to Bar Asian Influenza." The article was bylined by Bess Furman, who said:

> The Public Health Service today called a meeting for Monday to consider ways to prevent the spread of the influenza from the Far East to this country.
>
> Dr. Leroy E. Burney, Surgeon General of the service, said members of the Advisory Committee would attend the meeting on Influenza, which he appointed today.
>
> Dr. Burney listed the precautionary steps against the new type of influenza that has been sweeping Japan, the Philippines, Hong Kong, Sumatra, North Borneo, and other parts of the Orient.
>
> These preventative measures include providing samples of the virus that causes the Oriental influenza to United States vaccine manufacturers with a view to developing a vaccine against it.[23]

The writer labeled the epidemic as "new," "Far East," "Asian," and as "Oriental."[24] The framing of exotic and Far Eastern was perpetuated. The mention of a vaccine as a preventative measure was a frame that was now literally identified—vaccines could prevent influenza. The U.S. surgeon general had taken definitive action, a plan had been laid, and a vaccine would be developed. This type of reporting was very optimistic, with the influenza epidemic under control by the U.S. government. Furman said:

> As assurance to the public the Public Health Service stressed these factors: The disease thus far has been mild, with most cases having only three or four days of fever. The death toll in the Far East is not considered high in view of the large numbers stricken.
>
> Prompt treatment with antibiotics can prevent the bacterial complications that have been the cause of most of the fatalities in influenza outbreaks in this country, such as in World War I.
>
> Most communities have health departments that link a state-federal-international reporting system so that individual cases are quickly spotted.[25]

Furman's article retold the history of manufacturing and using influenza vaccines by the army. She reemphasized the optimistic approach to dealing with the threat of an influenza epidemic. The same day that Furman's article ran, a much smaller article, from Santa Ana, California, followed and said, "E. L. Russell, Orange County Health Officer, reported that two cases of influenza apparently similar to the Asian type were discovered here yesterday."[26] The Asian influenza virus was now making its debut in the United States.

The next day, a report from Australia said, "Australian scientists have developed a vaccine to combat an influenza epidemic sweeping the Far East from India to the Philippines."[27] The article explained that the epidemic was caused by a "mutant virus that sidesteps natural body defenses against normal influenza virus," and in order to establish immunity, "whole populations would require vaccination."[28] The framing used in this article placed emphasis on the need for vaccination in order to escape the potentially deadly effects of the flu. The same day, an editorial was run discussing the issues thus far framed about Asian influenza. The editorial outlined the current status and recent history of the epidemic:

> Health authorities in the United States and in Great Britain have warned that there is one likelihood that the disease will appear in this country and in Europe before the year is over. They add, however, that we need not expect or fear a repetition of the deadly epidemics of 1917 and 1918. But any disease that can quickly sweep over victims that number into the millions is a serious matter.
>
> Fortunately, also, we are better equipped to deal with such a problem than we have in the past. Already the special virus of this Asian variant of the influenzas has been identified and laboratories here and abroad are hard at work on the preparation of vaccines.[29]

Again, emphasis on the vaccination as a means to prevent contracting Asian influenza was reiterated. Even though the editor said that this strain was mild and death rates were low, there was still the potential for death. The editor ended the editorial with a discussion about the name, for which he attempted to reframe the foreign tag:

> This is another instance in which we can be made to realize that many health problems are truly world-wide and that world-wide action and cooperation are needed. It isn't just "Asian" influenza, although that name has already been pinned on it. It is a broadly human ailment that must be met wherever it appears.[30]

On the page after the editorial, the *New York Times's* science editor William L. Laurence wrote a story that said the 1957 epidemic was "the largest epidemic of influenza in years."[31] He retold the recent history of the disease and used a research scientist at the World Influenza Center in London as a source for the information. He reiterated, via scientific attribution, that the current virus was fairly mild and definitely much less dangerous than the Spanish influenza virus. In summarizing the article, Laurence said:

> The first human influenza virus was discovered in England in 1933 and was named type A. Type B was discovered in the United States in 1940. No one knows which type, if any, caused the epidemic of 1918. In fact, it is not definitely known whether the epidemic was actually influenza.[32]

Laurence did not attribute the "fact," but by saying this, he framed the Spanish influenza virus as possibly not influenza; therefore the Asian virus was possibly not related to the deadly predecessor. Essentially, even though many new stories had made a link or reference to the Spanish influenza, which had been acknowledged as killing twenty to thirty million persons, Laurence attempted to undo the link and framed Asian influenza as a virus that may not have a connection to its supposed deadly predecessor. This type of framing, while optimistic, began a trend that could be considered defensive in light of past history and news reportage.

The continued coverage of the Asian influenza epidemic then fell back on previous trends created by the Spanish influenza pandemic. First, reports began to track ships and planes carrying influenza-infected passengers to the United States. Then the involvement of public health officials and the possibility of quarantines arose, after which the spread of the epidemic across the United States was reported consistently and almost on a daily basis in the *New York Times*. However, a new frame emerged during the initial stage of infection in the United States in reference to vaccines. The frame evolved as a debate between public health recommendations and actual vaccine policies.

The framing of the vaccine debate continued to evolve. On June 11, 1957, the production of the vaccine was described, as was the surgeon general's decision to have all U.S. troops vaccinated before civilians.[33] A couple days later, the New York State Health Department announced a plan to combat influenza by starting a pilot project to produce a vaccine for Far East influenza.[34] The article was a reiteration of a statement from Governor Averill Harriman and Dr. Herman E. Hilleboe, the state health commissioner. According to the article,

> the department wanted to be prepared in case the disease should make a sudden appearance in this country.
>
> Governor Harriman, at a conference with Dr. Hilleboe today, authorized the Health Department to take whatever steps are necessary to deal with the arrival of the Far East strain of influenza in New York.
>
> A Health Department announcement explained that none of the influenza vaccines on hand in the United States was effective against the Far East strain.[35]

The article emphasized the need for a suitable vaccine and framed this need being met by the state health department, rather than by a federal agency.

While quarantines were being discussed among countries that had not yet been terribly affected, the WHO released a statement saying "quarantining could not stop the spread of influenza," and that "acute cases should be isolated, the United Nations agency recommended, but large-scale efforts at quarantining were termed 'as costly as they are ineffective.'"[36]

The WHO also emphasized the mildness of the disease by saying, "Very few deaths have been scientifically proved to be due to this cause and are mostly among elderly people suffering from chronic bronchitis." This statement used a device to frame science or scientific standards as an absolute in defining facts about influenza. The sentence also identified a high-risk group: older chronically ill persons. To date, deaths from Asian influenza had been identified with two high-risk groups: the elderly and school-age children.

In nonlocal international news by the *New York Times*, articles chronicled other countries' efforts to create a vaccine for their use. Both Great Britain and Australia said they had isolated the Asian flu virus and were testing effective rates.[37] The next day, the United States Public Health Service announced, "work on the new experimental vaccine for Oriental influenza now was in its clinical trial stage."[38] They also reported that volunteers had been inoculated and it would take about six weeks to determine whether antibodies developed, which would indicate an effective vaccine.

A couple of days later, reports of Asian influenza outbreaks among the navy appeared. In an attempt to explain how the navy was infected, the article said:

> One health officer said reports that the Navy men had not been in contact with persons from the Far East indicated the Oriental influenza possibly could have spread to the United States through Europe.[39]

In reference to a vaccine:

> About 100 laboratories are seeking to develop a vaccine for the new type of influenza. Public health officials feel that the United States will escape any serious epidemic if an effective vaccine is developed before fall.[40]

The framing of Asian influenza solidified the trend to put blame for the virus elsewhere and point a finger at a foreign introduction, rather than assume local responsibility. The framing of a vaccine was now seen as an international race to make an effective vaccine in order to save the United States from the injustices of another influenza epidemic.

On June 23, an in-depth story by Howard A. Rusk, M.D., presented an analysis of "the disease and steps scientists are taking for a vaccine."[41] Rusk literally described the framing of the Asian influenza virus to date:

> Fortunately, for a variety of reasons, this epidemic will not take a toll in lives similar to that of 1918–1919. In that pandemic, about 20,000,000 people died. More than 12,000,000 persons died in India alone, and 548,000 in the United States.
>
> There are reasons for optimism in the current situation.
>
> First, the virus causing the disease in the current epidemic is fairly innocuous with most cases having only three or four days of aches and fever. Deaths have been limited and have occurred primarily among young children and very old people.
>
> Second, although there is no specific treatment for the influenza, once it is contracted, the dangerous complications such as bacterial pneumonia can be controlled by antibiotics and sulfa drugs.
>
> Third, if the disease reaches the United States in serious proportions, vaccine to combat it should be commercially available.[42]

The next day, Merck, Sharp, and Dohme, a Philadelphia pharmaceutical company, announced that it had successfully produced laboratory quantities of a new vaccine for the Asian flu and would "produce the vaccine on a large-scale basis should conditions warrant."[43] The vaccine was being tested by the National Institutes of Health (NIH), the article continued. While the notion that a suitable available vaccine was on the horizon for Americans, another article, which would be referred to more often than any other article prior to the actual pandemic, was run on June 26.[44]

Dr. Leroy E. Burney, surgeon general of the Public Health Service, announced that the "spread of the disease to this country is regarded as highly likely," and

> reports from the Far East to date indicate that, although the attack rate is high, running from 15 to 20 per cent of the population in the affected countries, the mortality rates are low.[45]

The primary rhetorical framing device that was pulled from this story and repeatedly used was that the United States was going to be infected by the Asian influenza epidemic with a 10 to 20 percent infection rate.

Reports of the spread of influenza across Europe continued, while the Far East began its recovery.[46] In the United States, the *New York Times* reported that six American pharmaceutical companies announced that they had "perfected a low-cost vaccine against Asian influenza."[47] The only snag in mass-producing the vaccine was that the NIH had to "establish standards for manufacturing procedure, potency and safety" and authorize the mass-production.[48] On July 10, the Public Health Service made its "first official confirmation of the appearance of Asian influenza among civilians in this country."[49] Again, scientific rhetoric was attached to facticity regarding influenza in the announcement when it stated: "The virus attacking a girls' group in Davis, Calif., was shown by laboratory tests to be the new flu that has swept many countries in the Far East." The article said that the Asian influenza virus had already been noted among armed forces personnel at Newport, Rhode Island; Norfolk, Virginia; and San Diego, California. The article ended with a prediction that "by October a vaccine against the disease will be made available to the public."[50]

The next day in another announcement, the Public Health Service said it "had established specifications for the manufacturer of vaccine containing the new Far Eastern influenza strain."[51] However, there was no mention of how much vaccine would be made and by when.

The first significant outbreak reaching epidemic proportions was reported by the *New York Times* on July 27, when twelve thousand cases with four deaths were reported in San Diego, California.[52] Seven thousand of the cases were military personnel, but the four deaths were civilians. The article ended by stating that "Admiral Gillett declined to say if the Navy believed that the disease might have been brought to this city aboard ships returning from the Orient."[53] Again, there was an attempt to attach the influenza epidemic to a foreign locale, but this time, it appeared that officials declined to feed into this type of framing.

The next day, the American Medical Association (AMA) told the press that a nationwide preparedness program had been initiated and "stressed that there was 'no immediate cause for alarm.'" The AMA spokesperson then estimated that the rate of attack "'would run between 15 and 20 per cent of the population of any cities where the disease reached epidemic proportions.'"[54] The article, both in headlines and text, basically "put the United States on alert," and then reversed itself rhetorically by saying there was no need for alarm.[55] This double-sided message began a period of moving the framing of the Asian influenza pandemic from optimistism to defensive optimism.

An editorial on July 31 presented a more optimistic view of Asian influenza, invoking war rhetoric in order to calm any perceived anxieties:

> Since the early outbreaks there has been a steady effort to provide a good means of immunization. Thus far good results have been achieved and further progress can be expected. The virus has been identified and *combative* sera have been developed. It is unlikely that a nation-wide campaign will be required, but if it is, there will be the *weapons* for it at hand.
>
> Meanwhile, the best medical advice is to *be on the lookout* for any respiratory complaint. If it appears it should be promptly reported and *countermeasures* taken. We do not face the awful dangers of the epidemic of 1918–19, but we face a troublesome *enemy* to our well-being and, fortunately, we can do something about it.[56] (Emphasis mine.)

As news of a vaccine spread, stories turned to framing the vaccine instead of influenza. How the vaccine was actually manufactured and when it would be available emerged as two major framing devices. The first article to begin using these devices was run on July 31 in the *New York Times*.[57] The article originated in Washington and was accompanied by a byline, "By Science Service."[58] This was the first article with this type of byline. In the body of the article, while the information is medical-technical information regarding vaccine production, there are no sources attributed. The article also said, "The first vaccine is expected to be ready by Aug. 15."

On August 2, 1957, an article by Bess Furman, out of Washington, said:

> The Public Health Service warned today of "the very definite probability"—not just a possibility—of a very large outbreak of Asiatic influenza in the United States this fall or winter. Surgeon General Leroy E. Burney voiced the prediction at a news conference. . . .
>
> "Undoubtedly," he said, "there is very wide seeding of the virus throughout the country."[59]

And in reference to the influenza vaccine:

> It takes ten days to two weeks after the injection for enough antibodies to build up to give protection for one year.

> The 60,000,000 doses, Dr. Burney said, would immunize about one-third of the population of the country. . . .
> He is suggesting that as the vaccine becomes available priority should be given to "those whose services are imperative for the care of the sick and those needed to maintain other essential functions."
> He estimated doctors, nurses, hospital attendants, and practical nurses at about 3,000,000. He said essential workers in the communication, transportation, and utility industries would build up to about 12,000,000 the number who should receive earliest vaccinations.
> Dr. Burney pointed out that when triggered by adverse weather, the disease could sweep from San Francisco to Boston in four weeks, incapacitating from 10 to 20 per cent of the population.[60]

This article framed influenza in a very serious manner. Despite emphasizing that the virus was mild in nature with few deaths, the surgeon general now warned American citizens that cities could be incapacitated by Asian influenza within four weeks of "seeding." Add to this that the virus was already spreading in the United States, only one-third of the population would receive a vaccine, and it takes time to build up immunities after receiving the vaccine; the result was that the framing of Asian influenza had switched from optimistic to the inevitability of going to war with an epidemic.

Dr. Leona Baumgartner, New York City's health commissioner, responded to Burney's warnings the next day and said:

> Medical authorities were making preparations to cope with any possible invasion of Asiatic influenza this fall or winter.
> Dr. Leona Baumgartner, the Commissioner, counseled residents "not to worry" about the "mild" disease.[61]

Regardless of the commissioner's "counseling," when a person was told not to worry, he or she worried. Asian influenza was now solidly framed in responding to the public's anxiety about contracting the flu. Additionally, if one suspected Asian flu, laboratory tests, which took up to two weeks to process, had to be run to confirm. Therefore, whether there was an actual outbreak, reports continued to follow "suspected" outbreaks of influenza, similar to tracking a hurricane without any real facts or up-to-date information.[62] Essentially, the hurricane could become destructive before there was actual confirmation of its path.

On August 8, 1957, a story from Washington said that President Eisenhower was seeking funds to help fight the flu and that the vaccine output was being sped up.[63] Several of Dr. Burney's remarks were restated in this article, as well as the mention that the armed forces would be receiving four million vaccinations, which was half of the first batch to be released:

> A goal of at least 60,000,000 doses by Feb. 1 has been set. This would be enough to vaccinate a third of the population of the United States, which was estimated by the Census Bureau at 171,000,000 on June 6.[64]

In order to reframe or console anxieties related to influenza fatalities, the article also said:

> The Health Service says such antibiotics as penicillin could be used effectively to combat pneumonia or other diseases that might strike as an aftermath of flu, although they have no value in fighting flu itself.
>
> Medical sources say that most of the deaths in the great flu epidemic of 1918–1919, which killed 20,000,000 persons, including 548,000 Americans, were attributable not to the flu itself but to bacterial pneumonias that often accompanied the disease.[65]

The next day, a local story reported that pharmaceutical houses were speeding up vaccine production and that in New York City

> possible symptoms of the mild disease have been detected in eight high school pupils from foreign countries who arrived by air Wednesday from Amsterdam, according to Dr. Roscoe P. Kandle, Acting Health Commissioner. . . .
>
> He said it would take several days before tests would show whether their illness was the result of the virus or of something else.[66]

The last paragraph of the article reported that "in another development, sixteen American delegates to the International Youth Festival at Moscow were reported to have been stricken with mild cases of influenza."[67] The framing of this story substantiated initial reports of influenza, placing the emphasis of blame for infection on foreign individuals or countries. A follow story was printed the next day to report that the foreign students were doing "very well."[68] Beneath this article a story from Geneva read:

> Asiatic influenza has traveled around the world in less than five months. The World Health Organization today reported outbreaks in South America, the last remaining continent to be affected.[69]

The Asian flu had officially reached pandemic proportions. What followed in the news coverage prior to the actual beginning of the flu season were both offensive and defensive stances in reference to vaccination. The federal government pushed for a national campaign to urge Americans to be vaccinated (offensive), while local governments struggled with how they would prioritize and vaccinate one third of their population (defensive). With each news story, a different public health policy was suggested, and in some cases, the stances of offensive and defensive frames switched places. Regardless, the news coverage presented a debate between city, state, and federal agencies over how vaccinations were going to be handled.

While the federal government advocated a national campaign urging the public to get shots,[70] it also called for a prioritizing in vaccinations, with the military first, populous areas second, and then essential workers within populous areas last.[71] Essentially, the federal government placed the responsibility on how the civilian population should be dealt with squarely on the shoulders of local public health officials. This responsibility was not an easy one to bear, especially when the surgeon general was practically guaranteeing an epidemic, that the vaccine would not be available until the middle of the influenza season, that only one third of the population could be vaccinated, and that one third now included the military. To frame the situation bleaker, in an August 13 article, after the surgeon general discussed his ideas for prioritizing vaccines, he said "even with the maximum use of the vaccine, this country may have serious influenza epidemics in the fall or winter."

The next day, the first page-one story with a large photo ran in the *New York Times*.[72] The photo was of the New York City Health Department's Bureau of Preventable Diseases Director Dr. Morris Greenberg examining several foreign students, who had recently arrived from Rotterdam, with suspected cases of influenza. In a separate article the framing of influenza and influenza vaccines was literally elaborated by Farnsworth Fowle:

> Every new contagious disease that looms over the city's horizon is a test of the Health Department's professional skill and practical judgment. It has drastic powers corresponding to its heavy responsibilities to protect the city's health.
>
> Asiatic influenza is a newcomer on this continent. The Health Department had previously set up an advisory committee to develop policy on the illness. A vaccine has been developed, but it is in too short supply for city-wide inoculation.[73]

What followed was a profile of Dr. Greenberg and a detailed explanation of his policies on quarantining ill foreign passengers. Fowle explained that Greenberg was practicing when the 1918 flu pandemic hit New York City, and that he (Greenberg) was very wary and cautious about making any "snap judgments."[74] This article is rare among the other stories. In framing influenza and the response from local authorities, the profile used a personnel narrative profile format to explain a public health policy decision. Greenberg, Fowle said, let all but twenty-seven students go on to their final destinations. The twenty-seven remaining students were kept aboard the ship because "none of the patients was sick enough to need immediate hospitalization."[75] Unfortunately, the newspaper reported the next day that one of the students had died and that "Asiatic illness" was suspected.[76] This was the first reported death from Asian influenza in New York City, although the report was not yet confirmed.

Of course, with a death now reported, the vaccine debate ensued. The response from New York City was that all "essential city service workers" were to be vaccinated before the general public, and local public health officials would leave it up to physicians to decide who would be vaccinated next.[77] The shift in responsibility was again reframed, with vaccines moving from a general or federal public health responsibility to an individual responsibility.

On August 18, a very optimistic story by Robert K. Plumb ran about Asian influenza that focused on scientific information and told that the influenza virus vaccine had been found to be only 70 percent effective.[78] Plumb also reiterated that the fatality-causing effect of influenza was bacterial pneumonia, not the influenza virus, and pneumonia could be treated with penicillin. He recommended "priority in receiving inoculations against Asiatic 'flu' should be given to those who perform essential work, including the care of the sick."[79]

An editorial run the same day as Plumb's story restated that Asiatic flu was an "innocuous disease" whose potentially dangerous side effects could "be controlled by administration of antibiotics and sulfa drugs."[80] These stories illustrated an attempt to allay public anxiety over who should and should not be vaccinated and that the disease could be fought with readily available drugs. The next day, in a *New York Times* news story, Bill Becker covered New York Governor Harriman's appearance on WABD-TV. In the later part of the television program, Becker reported, the governor said that the "production of a vaccine for Asiatic flu was moving ahead and 'a considerable supply' would be available by October."[81] On August 20, an article from Washington reported that "the Senate passed a $1,824,001,547 supplemental appropriations bill" to include a project to fight Asiatic flu.[82]

A couple of days later, a local story ran about New York City's plan to purchase 200,000 vaccines for key municipal workers, such as firemen and policemen. The article stated:

> Thus far no general inoculation program has been set up in the city and health officials have urged private citizens to ask their doctors about the possibility of getting the vaccine.[83]

Toward the end of the article, it was said that hospitals had already ordered and received vaccinations for their employees. This article had now framed the responsibility of vaccination on the individual. It appeared that employers of "essential" employees, especially city and state employees, had taken care to have them vaccinated. The general public, it appeared, had been left to fend for themselves. This shift in framing, from public health to individual health, marked the general shift in public health policies and philosophies as a whole.

On August 24, 1957, an article from Washington stated that the new influenza would be called Asian influenza, as per the surgeon general.[84] Therefore, in print, and in the United States, the Asian influenza pandemic was officially defined by its present-day name. The next day, the surgeon general announced that any persons allergic to eggs should "pass up Asian flu shots" and that for "all others in all age groups the vaccine 'is recommended.'"[85] It is interesting to note that the federal government, via the surgeon general, was still advocating that all persons, except those with egg allergies, get vaccinated, despite the fact that all persons were not able to do this due to a shortage in available vaccines. Therefore, while local stories tried to frame vaccination as unnecessary, the federal government maintained widespread inoculation, despite the fact that this was not possible.

On August 27, a page-one story by W. H. Lawrence reported that President Eisenhower was inoculated against Asian flu, despite the fact that "the President was reluctant to take the inoculation while supplies were limited and not generally available to the public."[86] Further down in the story, Lawrence attributed Dr. Burney with saying, "persons with a history of heart or lung ailments should be inoculated early" and stated, "Dr. Burney told Dr. Snyder there was an adequate supply of vaccine in the Washington area to take care of this group." This is the first time that the influenza vaccination was framed to identify a high-risk population as eligible for "priority inoculation."[87] This type of frame in this particular story signified a change in public health policies during the Asian influenza pandemic. To date, reports of fatalities had mentioned the very young, the aged, and the chronically ill, but policies reported by media up until then had not framed high-risk as a consideration for priority inoculation.

The next day, a headline read "Flu Shot Priority Set For City Aides" for New York City.[88] According to the article, Mayor Robert Wagner, of New York City, made an official announcement regarding the city's policy for Asian flu inoculation. The system consisted of inoculating in order of priority: doctors, nurses, policemen, and firemen. After these groups were inoculated, vaccines could be offered to employees in health clinics; workers in the medical examiner's office; child-care workers for institutions and shelters; utilities, communications, and emergency services personnel; and then teachers, day-care staff, and similar group caregivers.[89] This article reestablished the frame of inoculation for essential service employees first. Children, the elderly, or chronically ill, those already identified as the majority of the fatalities, were not included in the actual priority policy for New York City.

On August 29, it was reported that pharmaceutical companies were attempting to produce more doses of vaccines than had originally been anticipated, which might allow for the vaccination of almost half the population sometime in January 1958.[90] Dr. William Stewart, assistant to the surgeon general, warned, "'People need to know that there is not going to be enough vaccine for everybody for a while, and those who take care of us while we are sick or provide essential community services should get the vaccine first.'"[91] However, the article stated that Dr. Stewart recommended that "patients with such chronic diseases as heart ailments, diabetes and tuberculosis" should be vaccinated after hospital personnel.[92]

The same day, the issue of how long the flu shot would protect an individual was presented for the first time.[93] The article said that the immunity from a vaccine was approximately three to twelve months, but no one would really know for sure until there was wide use.[94] While adding more ambiguity to the framing of the flu vaccine, the article did establish that flu vaccines were not new:

> In almost every year since 1933, when the influenza virus was first discovered, there had been a recorded epidemic of flu somewhere in the world. In one important respect, however, the outbreaks of Asian flu this year have been different. . . .
>
> [T]he new vaccine is not much different from influenza vaccines that have been in use since 1941, according to a virus expert.[95]

News coverage now emphasized that people around the world were being affected and that the Asian epidemic was reaching pandemic proportions.

At the end of August, a new frame for Asian influenza appeared with a new set of arbiters: insurance companies and the call for sick persons to not go to the hospital.[96] According to author Peter Kihss:

> The advice of a top insurance medical official is to stay home instead of going to a hospital if you come down with Asian influenza. Health insurance may not cover the medical bill, but a patient is more likely to escape secondary infections from outside contacts.
>
> "We're not trying to dodge responsibility, but you're better off at home," says Dr. George M. Wheatley, third vice president of the Metropolitan Life Insurance Company.[97]

Prior to this article, the only advice for a person who actually got sick was "bed rest and a bland diet."[98] The insurance company advocated vaccination to prevent its policyholders from becoming ill. The insurance company was advocating the same preventative policies, but it was introducing yet another frame, which dictated that being in the hospital might be more dangerous to one's health than being at home. This frame brought about a new response from public health professionals during September, which was to not only place responsibility for vaccination with the individual, but for each household to send a person to Red Cross training in order to assist medical professionals and their own households.[99]

Editorials by the *New York Times*, four in one day, summed up the framing of Asian influenza prior to the onset of the pandemic. Two editorials dealt with the arrival of influenza from across the ocean and how air travel had increased the speed of infection.[100] The next editorial dealt with the problem of not having enough vaccine, and the last editorial focused on calming anxieties, claiming there was "no reason to panic." The editorial reiterated that the Asian flu epidemic was mild with a 1 percent death rate, and, because of scientific advances, the country had antibiotics that could ward off fatal complications.

> Complications arising from Asian flu, primarily pneumonia will most likely occur only among the very young, aged, and infirm; and these, unlike those of thirty-nine years ago, can be cured with the new wonder drugs and antibiotics.[101]

The last sentence in the editorial, however, reiterated anxieties about obtaining a vaccine, and said, "Only the vaccine, however, can stop Type-A Variant—the omnipotent intruder."

The paradox in the editor's composition is noteworthy. Was it sarcastic? The context of public health framing so far was that essential workers must be vaccinated before any high-risk groups. The editor pointed out which were the high-risk groups and then signified the vaccine as "omnipotent." Given the general nature of editorials to criticize public policies, one could assume that the editor was aware of the framing and chose to point out, in an ironic fashion, the blatantly obvious: those who were dying were not receiving vaccines.

Several days later, in a letter to the editor on September 6, one physician pointed out the potential problem in not having enough vaccine for those who wanted it, and that perhaps the policy to have the physician as the middle man for public health administration was not a fair one. He said:

> With the announcement of a protective vaccine against disease and with a forecast that there may not be enough of this material to go around before that epidemic may strike, apprehension has grown in many people who fear they may not be able to receive the vaccine in time from their physicians. . . .
>
> By what standard shall the physician determine who is to receive the vaccine when the first limited supply becomes available?

> Would it not be better for orderly administration of the vaccine by health agencies, using it for entire groups at a time, as it becomes available until the private physician can obtain all he requires for his patients?
>
> Could not such advertised procedure serve as a guide for future discoveries of this sort, so that mass anxiety neuroses are avoided, a situation that occurred at the time of the polio vaccine as well?[102]

The letter was anonymously signed M.D. and brought to the forefront the potential for problems with public health policies under the current system in place. The shift in framing from a public health issue with the responsibility of the federal government to state, to city, to physicians, to individuals, appeared to be a shift in policy that was not well received at the time.

The news coverage for the rest of September 1957 in the *New York Times* gradually brought to the forefront a public health debate, which had, up to then, been an undercurrent in influenza framing by the media. The debate ensued between national, state, and local public health authorities. On September 7, the American Medical Association (AMA) warned that the use of antibiotics with influenza patients was "not just worthless, but was dangerous."[103] It also backed up the insurance companies and said that "in its uncomplicated form," victims of influenza were better off at home.[104] The AMA said that no antibacterials or antibiotics should be used as preventatives to influenza, and only in the case of secondary bacterial infections should antibiotics be used.

Two safeguards framed by local public health officials had been the use of antibiotics and hospitals. After all, hospital employees had been vaccinated and were ready to accommodate sick people, and there was plenty of penicillin to go around. The next day an article ran in which the American Red Cross, out of Washington, said, "Every family in America should arrange now for at least one member to take the Red Cross home nursing course."[105] The forty-hour course, the Red Cross said, would train family members to assist doctors and nurses. In another article on the same page, a "Flu Discussion" was covered in which "a panel of city health experts agreed that there was 'no reason for alarm.'"[106] The article also said:

> Asked why the vaccine was manufactured if the disease were not expected to be serious, Dr. Greenburg said it could affect 20 per cent of the population. He pointed out that if some city departments—such as hospitals and police—were undermanned for a few days, it would interfere with the city's necessary services.[107]

This type of framing suggested the presence of criticism in reference to public health policies and that the public *was* very anxious about the possibility of an influenza epidemic. (Emphasis mine.)

The next day, the *New York Times* ran a state priority list for flu shots with the story originating in Albany, New York.[108] The state health department essentially reiterated what the New York City Health Department had issued. However, immediately following the story, another story without a headline:

> A similar schedule of priorities among municipal employees was announced here on Aug. 27 by Mayor Wagner. It will be followed in administering the 200,000 shots of vaccine ordered last month for city employees.[109]

This aside emphasizes the fact that New York City had already adopted its own public health policy and would be using it instead of the state's policy. This type of narrative suggests that the New York State and city officials were not working together.

The following day, September 11, a story by Layhmond Robinson ran from Washington, in which a summary blurb stated, "Experts Deny Conflict With Surgeon General's Views on Mass Inoculations."[110] The article said:

> The Health Department's advisory committee on influenza declared yesterday that it did not know enough about the effectiveness of Asian influenza vaccine "at this time" to urge its use by the general public.
>
> Although the committee members vigorously denied it, their statement appeared to conflict with the recommendations by Dr. Leroy E. Burney, the United States Surgeon General, that as many persons as possible be inoculated with the vaccine as soon as it became available.[111]

Now there was discord among national and local officials. Robinson said the committee decided that essential workers should be vaccinated, but, as Robinson points out, "but neither in their statement nor at a later press conference did committee members explain what they meant by 'essential workers.'"[112]

Two days later, the state health department reiterated its support for mass inoculation, supporting the surgeon general.[113] The article then restated that the New York City Health Department had a problem with ascertaining whether the flu vaccine was effective and was reluctant to advocate mass inoculation. The state spokesman said, "We believe the new vaccine is effective" and "We have no evidence that it is less effective than vaccines that have been used against other types of influenza."[114] This type of framing reemphasized the discord in public health policy during the Asian flu epidemic in New York State. The next day, September 14, another article by Layhmond Robinson reported that New York City had taken a "neutral" position in reference to mass inoculation and that a "departmental advisory committee needed more time to evaluate the new Asian influenza vaccine before urging it for general public use."[115] Robinson reiterated that the surgeon general and state health department had both urged mass inoculation.

Following this article was an article initiated by the WHO from "United Nations, N.Y.," which said:

> The current "panic" caused by the Asian influenza epidemic represents an unrealistic attitude, according to a report issued today by the World Health Organization. The epidemic is actually very mild, the report said, and should be no cause for alarm.[116]

Again, the stories were consistent with a frame of discord among the general public and public health professionals. The next day, a large story containing eight small stories from "New York suburbs" illustrated the disconnection among public health officials by presenting "priority lists" from several areas around New York City.[117] Each list, from Nassau, Suffolk, Westchester, Rockland, Hudson, and Bergen, New Jersey, and New York City, contained a different prioritized list that categorized who should be vaccinated first. One story from Trenton, New Jersey, reported, "a bill was scheduled to be introduced in the New Jersey Legislature, which convenes Nov. 18, to make the vaccine available to all municipalities in the state."[118]

While the effectiveness of the vaccine was debated, priority lists drawn up, and vaccines distributed, a report from London said that two British warships had come down with Asian influenza and had to cancel their North Atlantic Treaty Organization (NATO) exercises with American warships.[119] The article also pointed out that the "more than 85,000 American officers and men were inoculated against the disease before the ships left their home ports," and that none of the Americans had contracted the disease so far. This translated as a 100 percent effective rate for the Asian influenza vaccine, but it was not reported that way, only framed that way. The article immediately following the London report, by Bess Furman, said, "Asian influenza spread faster than teams of experts could be sent in to record its sweep" and Dr. Fred L. Soper, director of the Pan American Sanitary Bureau, said:

> Not a sign of the disease was present, he said, when one of his teams visited Chile in mid-July. In ten days, there were 2,000,000 cases. More than 1,000,000 persons were afflicted in a population of 6,7000,000 during the few weeks that the epidemic raged.[120]

The article also reported the death rate was "far more severe for those over 55 years of age," and that there were almost "no deaths among children under 10."[121] The article ended with a quote from Dr. Soper, who said, "Despite reports of its mildness, Asian influenza hit the individual 'all over' and should be avoided if possible."[122] Again, there is an emphasis on the severity of the disease, and, while it does not kill many people, it strikes suddenly and should be avoided. With this type of framing, the vaccine was the only thing that could stop the "omnipotent intruder" that the *New York Times* editorial said the Asian influenza was.[123]

The next day an editorial ran that returned to an optimistic outlook and heralded scientific advancements that allowed for a quick vaccine and antibiotics to ward off any evil complications. The editorial concluded:

> Meanwhile, we can all be proud of the early discovery of the new type A virus in Asia, quick development of a vaccine against it, and extensive medical record-breaking of the spread of the disease—all are evidence of man's improved ability to cope with virus diseases. Of these, influenza has usually been the mildest.[124]

The editorial framed science as if it were trying to place faith in science instead of God. Its optimistic outlook reiterated the earlier frames begun by the *New York Times*, but perhaps panic and anxiety had already taken hold. Over the next several weeks, the Asian flu began to sweep the United States. By September 14, it had already reached epidemic proportions in Louisiana. On September 19, New York City decided to endorse mass inoculation, and key civil service workers were inoculated against Asian influenza.[125] On September 20, the state health department for New York estimated "suspected cases of Asian influenza in New York had risen to 1,162 in eighteen separate outbreaks," and more than 100,000 flu cases had been reported in the United States.[126]

On September 25, 1957, the Public Health Service announced that it had "asked manufacturers of Asian flu vaccine to follow the priority recommendations of state and local advisory committees in filling orders" and recommended that "vaccinations be given first to those needed to care for the sick and to maintain essential services and to patients listed as high medical risks."[127]

The allocation of vaccinations, previously framed as a concern of the federal government via the surgeon general, was now in the hands of local authorities. The article announcing the allocation policy was attributed to the Public Health Service, but not to the surgeon general. With a shift in responsibility, there was a shift in arbiters. Now, the burden of responsibility for a major public health catastrophe was in the hands of local authorities. It is also interesting to note that "patients listed as high medical risks" was now officially framed by the media. By the end of September, outbreaks of epidemic proportions were being reported with regularity across the United States.

Meanwhile, the coverage leading up to the Asian flu pandemic in *The Times* (London) was considerably less frequent than in the *New York Times*. However, the framing of coverage by *The Times* was almost identical to the overall frame of the spread of the disease. Nonlocal coverage chronicled the spread of influenza from Hong Kong through the Far East, beginning with the first story on April 17, 1957.[128] The stories were short and to the point, emphasizing those infected in Far Eastern countries. It wasn't until May 31, 1957, that *The Times* began to report on local precautions. The timing of Great Britain's response to the possibility of a local epidemic correlates to the United States response.[129] The article, written by the anonymous "Medical Correspondent," emphasized that the Far East influenza was a "new" strain and that there was "no available vaccine."[130] It also pointed out a link to the past. However, the approach to the influenza vaccine was significantly different in Great Britain. The correspondent wrote:

> Although the W.H.O. official has expressed the view that "there is no cause for alarm," there must inevitably be comparisons with the serious epidemic which swept the world in 1918–1919. This also started in a mild form, but suddenly the virus assumed a more virulent form and the disease assumed a correspondingly more serious form.
>
> The fact that the present epidemic has spread so far without assuming a serious form does give grounds for hoping that it will remain so, but the public health authorities will need to keep a careful watch on the situation. Unfortunately, in view of the totally different nature of the infecting strain of virus, there is no available vaccine, nor would it be possible to produce one in sufficient amounts or in sufficient time to be of any use should the epidemic cross the Channel within the next few weeks.[131]

The significant difference in framing by the British, as opposed to the United States, was clearly different in the approach to the vaccination issue. The British, at the onset, pointed out that even though a vaccine would be beneficial, the circumstance and timing made it impossible to expect one. In contrast, the *New York Times*, via the surgeon general, insisted that a vaccine was the only safe sure thing to do and emphasized what was attempting to be done. The framing of the vaccine situation in the *New York Times* was simply not logical.

On June 5, a warning from the WHO was run and ended by saying, "Officials said that attempts were being made in Britain and in the United States to cultivate the virus and produce a vaccine on a large scale."[132] The next day, in a written reply, *The Times* (London) ran an article that stated in the headline, "Precautions Taken."[133] In this article, the minister of Health essentially said that a reporting system had been put in place to track the epidemic both internationally and locally, and that "practitioners are now being reminded of these arrangements."[134] The minister also emphasized that the new flu was "clinically mild in nature."[135] From the British standpoint, the vaccine or scientific advancements were not framed optimistically.

On June 10, it was reported that Australian scientists had "evolved a vaccine to combat the influenza virus which is active in Asia, and mass production had begun."[136] (The *New York Times* reported the same information the day before.)[137] The same day, an article reported that a ship had come into the Tilberry port with reports of eighty-six cases of influenza among the crew and passengers, but the ship was given normal clearance by port health authorities, the article said.[138] This emphasized the frame of "no alarm" as opposed to the United States approach, which presented detailed coverage of any infected foreigners arriving by air or sea.

A couple of days later it was reported by the medical correspondent that Swedish and Australian laboratories had begun to manufacture vaccines.[139] However, while there was mention of a priority system for inoculation being set up in Australia, similar to what the United States was doing, the framing of the article was different. Sir John Charles, the chief medical officer of the Ministry of Health, was quoted to have said:

> It is unlikely that the vaccines, which have been prepared against past influenza strains, will protect against the infection by the new variant, and the possibilities of preparing a vaccine against the recently isolated strains are being actively explored. However favourably this work might proceed, there would be an inevitable delay before such a vaccine could be produced in quantity.[140]

Again, the frame of not being able to produce a timely vaccine was reported by the British press. On June 17, *The Times* quoted an Australian health official who had recently arrived in London as saying that he thought the Asiatic flu would "cover the whole world."[141] He predicted that the flu would be in Britain by winter and said, "I think it will probably be fairly mild here, but it will certainly come."[142]

On June 18, an article reported that a vaccine for the Asiatic flu was developed "in the Department of Virus Research in the Wright-Fleming Institute of Microbiology in London, where penicillin was discovered."[143] The article also said that the first batch of vaccine would be available in two weeks, but how the vaccine would be used had not been decided. Another health official said that "authorities" might choose priority groups for vaccination.[144]

Next to the article was a report that the first case of "suspected" Asian influenza had been reported to British health authorities.[145] This was the first mention of penicillin with influenza stories, and it was not framed the same way it was in the *New York Times*. So far there had been no mention of scientific advancements nor the use of penicillin for secondary infections. The story of the first suspected case followed the vaccine information. It was not accompanied by much information, but it did point out that the first suspected case was a foreigner who had recently returned to London.

The first real signs of anxiety about influenza vaccines appeared July 2, 1957, in *The Times*.[146] The article was presented in a question and answer format with the British minister of health. The question: "There has been some anxiety that there might not be sufficient supplies of vaccine available should there be a large number of cases: could an assurance on that point be given?" The minister of health replied that the vaccine was being produced and tested on a "laboratory scale," and "it should not be assumed, in view of the rather mild nature of the disease, that vaccination would necessarily be appropriate."[147]

The reportage reiterated that the British government was not advocating mass inoculation, but was emphasizing the mild nature of the new strain. A week later, an article reported a session in the "House" where a question was posed to the "government" about the measures being taken against Asian influenza.[148] The Earl of Onslow replied that there was no indication of spread, even though there were confirmed cases, and that again, "it should not be assumed that vaccination would necessarily be an appropriate measure for general use."

A week later, influenza had reached epidemic proportions in Australia, and "vaccination of key workers in essential services is to begin immediately."[149] This was the first time that the term "essential workers," in reference to who should be vaccinated, was used in foreign coverage. While the term was identical to framing devices used in the *New York Times*, the article was only one sentence long and did not receive any more attention than any other "telegram in brief," even though Australia is a part of Britain's Commonwealth.

On July 18, 1957, a letter to the editor was run, which called for British authorities to "intensify precautions" in Great Britain.[150] The letter ended with a very strong appeal in reference to the previous pandemic. It said, "If this 'Asian' pattern bears any resemblance to that of 1919, instant action and widespread preventive action would appear to be called for."[151] Even though the frame presented by the British government was that the flu was mild and there was possibly no need for mass inoculation, it appears that the general public was still responding the same way as United States citizens, which was with extreme anxiety. The next day an article ran that said, "the virulence of the influenza virus might be altering," and "in view of what had been accomplished it would be unrealistic to visualize control of influenza with the immunizing agents they had." The article reiterated the frame that the vaccine might not be a practical solution.

An editorial on July 23 also reiterated that there "should be some comparisons with the serious epidemic which swept the world in 1918–1919, but such a comparison should not be carried too far."[152] Again, the Asian flu was downplayed into a frame of *serious, but not deadly*. (Emphasis mine.) Another article from Geneva ran a statement from the WHO that said, "The death rate remains on the whole negligible." The framing of the influenza outbreaks was presented in a manner to allay any perceived fears. The coverage then turned to detailing vaccine production and the efforts of local laboratories and the WHO.[153]

In a letter to the editor on July 31, titled "Influenza Pandemic," a doctor wrote that the government should take care to make sure backup physicians were available if family practice physicians were to become ill or overworked.[154] The physician framed the "pandemic" in an alarmist fashion, directly related to his personnel needs. He said, "In an epidemic the whole national insurance scheme would break down, but before that happened a great many lives would be lost simply because it would be quite impossible to examine patients."[155] The doctor explained that because doctors are already overworked by the current system in England, that in the case of an epidemic, there would be deaths not necessarily due to influenza, but due to neglect from the daily regular workload.[156]

On August 8, a letter to the editor appeared in which a health insurance authority said that in the case of an epidemic, they were prepared to modify public health policies.[157] This was a timely response to a potential problem, emphasizing the framing of addressing public anxiety and not sensationalizing information in the British press.

By August, it was reported that the British influenza vaccine for Asian influenza had been successfully tested and was now being produced in mass quantities. However, the director of the laboratory where the vaccine was being produced said:

> It remains to be seen whether the vaccine will give protection against Asian 'flu, but we won't know that until it comes. From inference we have good reason to believe that the vaccine will give protection. Meanwhile we are producing the vaccine, and hope that the first supplies will be on sale in shops within a month.[158]

The framing of the vaccine was neutral and "hopeful," while at the same time, the British government had not yet determined that vaccination was necessary.

By the end of August, influenza outbreaks in both the United States and Great Britain were being reported by *The Times*. On August 31, 1957, the

Ministry of Health issued a statement that acknowledged the outbreaks, but brought up the question of the effectiveness of the vaccine, saying, "Experience in past winters has shown that influenza vaccines have usually not given more than 30–40 per cent protection."[159]

This type of framing device was also used in the United States. The ministry also said, "There is on present evidence no medical necessity for general vaccination against an infection so mild in form, and indeed it would be very difficult" and "the question of offering vaccination to certain small priority groups exposed to special risks is under consideration."[160] The Ministry of Health had taken a neutral stance on the use of vaccines, and in all of its statements to the press, run by *The Times*, it had reiterated the frame that the virus was mild and a vaccine might not be necessary. The frame of prioritizing the vaccine for select groups had so far been very low-key in comparison to news coverage by the *New York Times*.

During the month of September, reports continued to chronicle the spread of influenza across Great Britain. The rhetoric of war was used with not as much flourish, but a story that ran on September 7 was interesting in that the term "seeded" was picked up by the WHO. Prior to this story, in which the WHO was detailing the spread of the virus, the United States surgeon general only used this terminology in print.[161] In the story, Great Britain was described as having been "well-seeded with Asian virus."[162]

The issue of a vaccine for the general public was laid to rest on September 12, when the Ministry of Health announced:

> Asian-type influenza, while highly infectious, is milder in character than the ordinary type of influenza to which we are accustomed. On present evidence there is no medical necessity for general vaccination against so mild a disease. On past experience the protection given vaccines of this type does not usually exceed 30–40 per cent.[163]

In reference to the framing of priority lists, the same article announced,

> The Government are, however, proposing to buy enough vaccine to offer vaccination to certain groups of doctors, nurses, and others who are specially exposed to infection and on whom any epidemic places an exceptionally heavy burden, such as general medical practitioners, hospital staffs, and local authority staff who care for the sick in their own homes.[164]

The article concluded, "[I]t is understood that all the vaccine needed for this purpose will be obtainable in this country." This type of reportage attempted to put an end to public anxiety by presenting this assertion and left almost no ambiguity to the framing of the British vaccine.

The vaccination narrative was not entirely put to rest, however, because on September 16 an article discussed an influenza outbreak on two Royal Navy submarines and said, "Firms wishing to obtain Asian influenza vaccine for their employees are being told that they must wait until those on the priority list for vaccination have been inoculated."[165] While a new idea that employers might be able to obtain vaccines for employees was being reported, it is interesting to note that when the *New York Times* covered the same story a day later, it reported that the British Navy was sick, NATO exercises were delayed, and none of the Americans in the exercises had come down with the Asian flu. This could be due to the framing of the vaccine as unnecessarily effective and unnecessary for the general population in the United Kingdom, while mass inoculation in the States was advocated. Had the London press run a report similar to the *New York Times*, the effectiveness of the vaccine would have been very evident and in opposition to the government's claim of a 30 to 40 percent effectiveness rate. In the following stories about the incident, the inoculation of American soldiers was not mentioned when discussing the sick British Navy men.[166]

Asian influenza reached epidemic proportions in Great Britain by mid-September, with fatalities being reported regularly. Articles chronicled the effects of the rapidly spreading virus, detailing school closings and businesses affected by absenteeism. However, the virus continued to be framed as "mild," even with a significant death toll in the same sentence.[167] While the infected and fatality counts rose, articles reported on the "early" distribution of vaccines to those on the government's priority list, with no apparent sarcasm or call for a mass inoculation.[168]

COVERAGE DURING THE PANDEMIC: OCTOBER 1957 THROUGH MARCH 1958

Early coverage of the pandemic during October 1957 in the *New York Times* consisted primarily of chronicling influenza outbreaks and responses to the outbreaks. By October 3, 1957, front-page coverage framed influenza at epidemic proportions in New York City.[169] On almost a daily basis, along with influenza coverage, the New York City Health Department ran a story titled "Instructions on Care of Flu."[170] The article debuted October first and ran during the first month of the pandemic, informing readers about influenza symptoms and treatment.[171] The article advised those who suspected they had the flu to "go to bed," and to call their doctor if their fever persisted for more than two days.[172] The article also said that if a sick patient could not reach his doctor, he "may call the emergency service of the county medical societies," and a list of telephone numbers followed.[173] This type of information emphasized the frame that influenza was considered a serious situation and that public health authorities would be available if normal medical channels were disrupted.

Nonlocal coverage was sparse during the height of the pandemic. On October 3, it was reported that Prince Charles, then eight years old, was sick with influenza.[174] A week later it was reported that Queen Elizabeth had been inoculated against Asian influenza.[175] Some coverage continued to frame the epidemic as severe and somewhat harsher than local coverage.[176] For example, it was reported that the Netherlands was experiencing 70,000 new cases each day.[177] On October 13, the *New York Times* reported "the Soviet Union nationalized the Asian flu" by choosing to call it the "Russian flu."[178] This illustrates that the framing of the definition of the Asian flu pandemic was not globally consistent.

During October, coverage varied between stories that emphasized an increase in cases and stories that reported death tallies but also reported that the flu was "mild."[179] This narrative framing was similar to the type of coverage during the Spanish influenza pandemic and represented conflicted anxieties about the occurring epidemic. To elaborate conflicting frames, one headline asked, "Is It a Real Epidemic?"[180] Robinson, the bylined author, wrote:

> Did New York City jump the gun on Asian influenza? Is the city in the grip of a real epidemic or a make-believe one?
>
> A behind-the-scenes dispute on these questions has broken out among some public health officials and virus disease experts in the city.[181]

Facts and frames of influenza coverage were reiterated, demonstrating conflicting frames. Robinson reported that, while there were large numbers of schoolchildren affected by influenza, he questioned why there were not reports of "absenteeism among workers in large business establishments."[182] However, the author reported both sides of the argument: the "doubters" and public health officials. The article ended with a reiteration of the vaccination narrative already established by earlier coverage. Robinson quoted a "high Health Department official," who said, "The question of whether you should take the vaccine has almost become academic. In the first place, everyone can't get it. In the second place, the epidemic might be over by the time it takes effect."[183]

Another debate erupted between physicians and business industries. Philip Benjamin reported that

> representatives of the medical profession complained yesterday that many physicians were being cut off from supplies of Asian influenza vaccine while industrial concerns were apparently receiving large amounts.[184]

This was the first time the vaccine was framed as a dispute between the medical and business communities. The medical community basically lost this fight when it was reported that "because of an 'over-all vaccine shortage,' first priority on the vaccine should be assigned to essential community workers."[185] After this need had been met, health authorities said the vaccine would be given to physicians, who then had to determine a priority system of their own, with an emphasis on "persons in ill health, to whom influenza might be fatal." The framing of responsibility for general public inoculation was placed directly on physicians in private practice.

In a letter to the editor the next day, one physician wrote:

> As is well known to the public, it is almost impossible for many people to get a prophylactic injection of virus vaccine by their private physicians. This is due to the fact that the suppliers of physicians, surgical supply houses and drug stores are unable to get the vaccine in any significant quantity.
>
> Where does the vaccine go? It goes, justifiably, to hospitals for their staff and personnel and to essential industries, but also to many nonessential enterprises, in order to keep business going.
>
> We private physicians receive many telephone calls daily from patients wanting injections. We have to tell them that we haven't got the material. We would like to give it to those patients who are suffering from heart disease, diabetes and other chronic ailments and for whom the contraction of influenza may be of serious consequences. They should have first priority in receiving the benefit of prevention of a disease which is harmless for the majority of the younger and healthy population.
>
> It is more important to preserve life than to protect business.[186]

The influenza vaccine narrative increased in intensity and importance, as reflected by an October 27 article picked up by the *New York Times* from a United Press Wire from Kansas City, Missouri. The article said:

> James Glayzer, 24 years old, was sentenced to one year and one day in prison yesterday for stealing Asian flu vaccine valued at from $15,000 to $20,000. Federal Judge Richard Duncan levied the term after declaring "anyone who would steal such a vaccine when there is such a terrific need for it, deserves no consideration."[187]

By mid-October, while high numbers of flu cases were framed as significant, the epidemic itself was framed as "waning."[188] On October 22, it was reported:

> High Officials of the Health and Hospitals Departments expressed private hopes yesterday that the city's mild epidemic of Asian influenza was past its peak.
>
> They warned, however, that the disease was hard to predict. An onset of bad weather could bring an upward turn, they said.[189]

This type of cautiously optimistic framing was a return to the initial coverage of the Asian influenza pandemic and was presented two days later in a page-one story. The national Public Health Service predicted that a "high and perhaps increased incidence of Asian influenza will continue for eight or ten weeks, at which time a decline is expected."[190] They also urged high-risk persons to be vaccinated in the next few weeks.[191]

By November 1, 1957, the impact of Asian influenza in the United States was being reported in most large cities, the Public Health Service said, and that the flu was waning.[192] However, just when optimism was making a comeback, the Public Health Service announced that a new "more powerful" vaccine would soon be available and that "many persons who have been vaccinated against Asian influenza should get a *second* shot."[193] (Emphasis mine.) Even though reports continued to cite a decline in infection and fatalities, a November 6 story from Washington introduced a new frame. The headline read, "Lethal Flu Epidemic Called New Threat" and the article was attributed to "a leading authority on influenza":

> The present epidemic of Asian influenza might be only the first wave of a more serious epidemic.
>
> Dr. Richard E. Schope of the Rockefeller Institute for Medical Research said a second wave might be as disastrous as the epidemic in the fall of 1918, which killed millions of persons.[194]

Dr. Schope said he "doubted that antibiotics would satisfactorily combat the bacteria that would accompany a second influenza wave."[195] This was one of the first truly alarmist frames for this influenza pandemic. A November 8 headline read, "Deaths From Flu Climb to 856 in U.S.," even though the Public Health Service reported in the story that the "percentage gain over the previous week was the lowest recently recorded."[196] While reports continued to chronicle the decline in Asian influenza infection rates and fatality rates, on November 10, a local story attributed the acting New York City health commissioner, who said, "the epidemic was not yet 'entirely over,'" and that "pregnant women 'most certainly' get two vaccinations."[197]

On November 15, 1957, a headline read, "Toll of Asian Flu Nothing Like 1918," and reported:

> The scientific watch on Asian influenza in the world this fall has provided no evidence of a world catastrophe like that of 1918 and 1919, when 20,000,000 people died of influenza and its complications.[198]

This was the second mention of the 1918 pandemic since the beginning of October. This article's narrative, however, is more optimistic than the other article, which was a call to alarm due to past historical experience. On November 17, to add to the frame of alarm based on the previous pandemic, a nonlocal story reported, "A second wave of Asian influenza is sweeping Japan and four deaths were reported in Tokyo today." The words "second wave" served as an alarmist framing device because during the 1918 pandemic, a second wave of influenza in 1920 proved to be just as fatal as the initial 1918 pandemic in the United States. The Spanish pandemic had already been framed prior to initial coverage, and a rhetorical connection to alarm was clearly indicated with this emerging theme.

However, just as quickly as a new alarm was framed, an optimistic frame countered. On November 22, a report from Washington by the Public Health Service said that there was a "national decline in Asian influenza."[199] Several "factors" listed emphasized that "the epidemic had passed its peak."[200] This type of narrative suggested that a sound argument was being made to illustrate that influenza was on the decline. In further reports, Asian influenza was framed as having met the "height of the outbreak, in mid-October."

Nonlocal coverage picked up the frame of the influenza epidemic being worse in a foreign country, but it also reiterated the rhetoric of a second wave on November 29. To illustrate the conflict in frames, a very telling headline on December 6 read, "Flu Severity Rises As New Cases Fall."[201] The body of the story said that New York health departments and hospitals reported no increases in severity for influenza cases. Therefore, while the information was framed as alarmist, the actual information reported was not.

The framing of a shortage of influenza vaccines for the general public changed when it was reported that, by the beginning of December, the supply of vaccines had exceeded the demand. The story ran in the business section of the paper and said, "Trade sources believe that unless there is an increase in the number of cases this winter it may be difficult for some of the drug concerns to come out ahead of their investments."[202] The framing of this story is similar to the frames that evolved at the end of the 1918 pandemic, in that financial concerns seemed to appear once public anxiety or illnesses declined.

Three days later, a story reported that 50 percent of the United States, or 82,000,000 patients, "cost the nation 282,000,000 'bed-days of disability.'"[203] The article attributed United States Surgeon General Burney in a speech delivered to insurance executives at an annual meeting in New York City. Dr. Burney also noted that department store sales "slipped 3 per cent, while drug store sales went up 10 per cent during this period."[204] Again, this type of framing was similar to the end of the 1918 pandemic; once lives were no longer at stake, financial concerns were framed.

Another frame similar to the 1918 pandemic emerged that reported statistics that gave the pandemic some definition or clarification in reference to the number of fatalities, those infected, and financial concerns.[205] In the body of the story, Dr. Burney warned "that further outbreaks" were still possible and cited the "'second wave' in Japan" as an example.[206] The article ended with Burney recommending that citizens continue to get vaccinated, as there were "22,000,000 to 25,000,000 doses still in the pipelines or on manufacturers' shelves."[207] This type of framing reiterated the end of a pandemic, with statistical information and financial information, but it also continued the frame established early on by the national government, which was one of alarm and a call for prevention via inoculation. On December 31, a report from the Public Health Service said that while there was "a continued drop in new cases of Asian influenza," "data showed that a second epidemic of Asian influenza in Japan had reached its peak in most areas."[208]

For the last three months of the pandemic, January through March 1957, news stories dropped off dramatically in the *New York Times*. This was unexpected, because as the stories that did run reported, a second wave of influenza hit the United States. On February 8, an article from Washington reported that the surgeon general was looking into "the cause of a steady rise in deaths from influenza."[209] Several days later, it was reported that "a second wave of Asian flu approached the epidemic stage" in Milwaukee.[210] Then on February 15, a report from Washington said "tests indicated any immunity conferred by Asian influenza vaccine disappeared in three months."[211] The framing of this particular article reiterated the potential need to be vaccinated, especially in lieu of a second wave, but the article ended by saying, "The service reported several other recurrences of Asian influenza but said 'no state reported any community-wide outbreak.'"[212]

The next day, a headline read, "Influenza Strikes Again in Cities," and the story was accompanied by an illustration that demonstrated that deaths from flu and pneumonia had increased for the months of January and February 1958.[213] The article said:

> The data led Dr. Burney to suspect that Asian influenza may be smoldering in other areas in the United States. This, he said, underscores the importance of second injections for elderly persons and others in special risk groups.[214]

The last sentence of the article said, "Similar observations were made during the great influenza epidemic of 1918."[215] This type of narrative is consistent with alarmist frames in the midst of a perceived threat. However, the framing of singling out certain groups as high risk had been reiterated and now established within the rhetoric of framing devices for influenza.

By mid-March, the Public Health Service began reporting again that there was a decrease in deaths from influenza and that there "was no evidence of community-wide influenza outbreaks now, though sporadic outbreaks continued."[216] By the end of March nonlocal news coverage had ceased, but on March 24, a new framing device for the Asian virus was initiated when it was reported that a new Asian variant of the virus that resembled "a strain noted in 1947–1956" was found in New York City.[217] The article also brought up the fact that the current available vaccine might not protect against the new variant. The next day, March 25, the Public Health Service said it had obtained samples of "a new and more virulent Asian influenza virus" from New York and was going to test it to ascertain "whether it is preventable by present influenza vaccines."[218] There were no more indexed articles for March in the *New York Times.*

Coverage by *The Times* (London) followed similar framing patterns, except public health debates were not framed as intensely as they were in the *New York Times* and magazine articles. In fact, quite the opposite happened. In an article on October 17, 1957, the headline read, "Influenza Epidemic 'Underestimated,'" and the article said:

> Recent comment in the Press had tended to underestimate the seriousness of the epidemic, which might well mean a deal incidence of 300 a million population, as in the influenza epidemic of 1951.[219]

This frame was new to the Asian pandemic and was nowhere present in coverage by the *New York Times*. One possible explanation for this could be the way *The Times* (London) did not question or bring issue with any public health policies that the Ministry of Health put forth. There was no coverage to negate any public health decisions. This article said the press was responsible for its neutral framing of influenza, not the Ministry of Health.

In other coverage, the same articles that ran in the *New York Times* about Prince Charles and Queen Elizabeth also ran in *The Times* (London), a day earlier in both instances.[220] The majority of stories simply covered available death statistics, and compared them to the previous year, illustrating that there was an increase in deaths from influenza during October.[221] On October 29, at the height of the epidemic in Great Britain, it was revealed that the Ministry of Health did not consider influenza a reportable disease and that it may take "five weeks or more to identify a particular influenza."[222] Therefore, both the press and the Ministry of Health were framed as underplaying the epidemic. In a sense, one frame nullified the other. This article also emphasized that

> the disease has been generally more apparent among schoolchildren and service men, but the Ministry point out that such an infectious illness naturally spreads more quickly and is more noticeable in Army camps or crowded classrooms, whereas there is no way of knowing how it may have affected women in their homes, for example. Summing up these imponderables, the Ministry cautiously venture the opinion that Asian influenza has not affected any age group in particular.[223]

The information in this article implied that there was really no identifiable high-risk group, which was contrary to news framing in the *New York Times*.

Beginning November 4, news reports began to chronicle the decline in Asian influenza cases and deaths.[224] Mid-January of 1958, an article reported that there was trouble with a staphylococcal infection in British hospitals, which might account for the 3,731 fatalities from influenza at hospitals.[225] According to the Public Health Laboratory service:

> the characteristics of the considerable number of deaths caused by the influenza virus. It caused sepsis, boils, and other conditions and led to trouble in hospitals because it had a way of becoming insensitive to penicillin and other antibiotics.
>
> Deaths often took place so quickly that treatment would probably have had no chance. . . .
>
> [T]he germ could kill within 24 hours. Once the influenza virus had paved the way and allowed the germ to multiply the patient turned blue and become asphyxiated.[226]

This information framed influenza fatalities not as a problem of underreporting or framing on behalf of the press or Ministry, but as a problem of an unexpected germ, whose timing was unfortunate. The article concluded, however, that this was not a new phenomenon:

> The appearance of staphylococcal infection is no new thing. In recent years during influenza epidemics, deaths have been associated with this staphylococcus.[227]

The last article during the pandemic time frame in *The Times* ran on February 15, 1958.[228] It was a nonlocal story from Geneva that said that the

> epidemic of Asian influenza affected about 12 million people in Britain, and was directly or indirectly responsible for about 16,000 deaths, the World Health Organization reported.[229]

AFTER THE PANDEMIC: APRIL 1958 THROUGH DECEMBER 1959

Coverage in the *New York Times* for the remaining months in 1958 was sparse and initially detailed statistics at the height of the epidemic.[230] At the end of May, new information was reported that suggested a more deadly strain of Asian virus had evolved.[231] On May 31, 1958, an article said:

> The city is studying the possibility that two influenza viruses have combined to form a new and more virulent strain. The possible new type may have developed from a combination of earlier strains and the Asian virus.
>
> News that such studies were in progress came to light following the publication of a laboratory analysis of the 1957–1958 outbreak of Asian influenza here. The analysis appears in *The Journal of the American Medical Association*.[232]

The frame introduced by this article was not that the virus had possibly mutated, which had already been established early on, but that the newspaper learned its information from a journal article that was revealed after publication. This is significant, because up to this point, all magazine or journal articles had previously advanced information to the media before actual publication. In fact, this was the first magazine article to report a different or new piece of information before a newspaper since the first magazine story in January 1957. The news article said that up to 35 percent of New York City had been affected by Asian influenza.[233]

On August 15 an article released from Geneva by the WHO said that "a new Asian influenza outbreak could be expected this year—but that it would be milder than the killer epidemic of 1957."[234] The WHO also said that the "Asian flu virus is lying dormant in millions of persons who act as its reservoir."[235] This type of framing of information was reminiscent of media coverage prior to the pandemic that served as an early warning system for worldwide public health concerns.

At the beginning of September, the national Public Health Service "recommended influenza shots for persons the disease might affect seriously."[236] This information reiterated a new public health policy that developed during the Asian influenza epidemic, which was that high-risk persons should be considered for inoculation first. The article ended with a warning from Dr. Burney that "any mass vaccination program should be begun before the influenza season."[237] The stance taken by Burney is also a new public health policy in that he was advising inoculation before the fear of a threat of influenza and before the start of the influenza season.

On September 24, the *New York Times* ran a story from the New York State Health Department, which said, "There is little likelihood that

Asian influenza or its allied viruses will strike a major blow at New York State this winter."[238] The framing of influenza here is interesting in that any new influenza threat was still being defined as "Asian," and that now, if the virus mutated, it was an "allied" virus. This type of rhetoric was consistent with the recent rhetoric of war, with a direct association to the allied forces, or NATO. The article is neutral in tone, because while it said not to expect a severe epidemic, "some influenza will be around." The framing of high-risk persons was reiterated toward the end of the article when the state health commissioner suggested that "persons susceptible to respiratory diseases and the chronically ill, the aged, and pregnant women should take the vaccine."[239] It was not until after this sentence that health-care workers, who had previously been a part of the priority elite, were now downgraded behind high-risk patients.

The last *New York Times* article for 1958 was a nonlocal story on November 21, which said, "Asian flu has struck again in Malaya. During the last two weeks 2,500 cases have been reported."[240] But, while the alarm had been raised, there was no new information of another epidemic until a January 4 article in Auckland, New Zealand.[241] The article said that a group of boy scouts was hospitalized after they contracted influenza at a Boy Scout Jamboree with 8,200 scouts present.[242] On February 7, a story ran that reported the surgeon general as saying that two new viruses had been isolated, which "cause illnesses similar to influenza."[243] Dr. Burney called this discovery "an important advance against one of our major public health problems."[244] This was the first time that influenza had been framed literally as a public health problem. Burney also said that the new viruses are more acute in hospitalized children and infants. This reiterated the frame that there were high-risk groups that were more prone to certain illnesses.

Nonlocal coverage in the *New York Times* picked up significantly during 1959, accounting for the majority of actual coverage, beginning with a flu epidemic that hit Great Britain.[245] An article on February 7, 1959, reported, "Britain continued to suffer today from four-day flu that many experts connect with the persistent fog." This was the first time in this study that London's fog was framed as a public health threat. The story also reported that Prince Charles, now ten years old, had come down with the flu at his boarding school.

Two days later, a story was released by the Public Health Service that said although no outbreaks of influenza had been reported in this country, the Public Health Service warned state health officers of increasing reports of flu outbreaks in Europe.[246]

The surgeon general said that an outbreak "was probable" in the United States, and that two students who had recently returned from

Norway had developed Asian influenza on the way back to the United States.[247] The article said:

> In England, the Asian strain of flu has been isolated from one fatal case and some other non-fatal cases. An epidemic of Type A influenza has been reported in the Soviet Union and Type B infections have been identified in Italy and the Netherlands.
>
> Mr. Burney again recommended that private physicians consider vaccinating individual patients or groups who have a special risk.[248]

The information in this article suggested that the United States surgeon general had a close watch on the world in reference to influenza. There was no mention of reports from the WHO to suggest otherwise. The article also demonstrated a sophistication of scientific knowledge about influenza in explaining the various strains. The frame of high-risk groups was also reiterated.

By mid-February, nonlocal coverage reported that in Great Britain "'everybody has got flu.'"[249] However, the type of flu the British had was not mentioned, only that it was mild and patients should "spend a few days in bed before calling in hard-pressed medical help." The next day two stories ran, one from a *Times* correspondent and one from the Reuters wire service, that differed greatly in their framing of the British influenza epidemic. The "Special to the *New York Times*" said:

> The death toll of the near-epidemic of influenza now sweeping England and Wales was 144 in the week ended Feb. 7. . . .
>
> Cases of other respiratory ailments also went up sharply.[250]

The information in this article suggested that the epidemic was severe and fatal in England. However, in the Reuters article, right after the first article, it said:

> Influenza is again sweeping Europe but outbreaks are reported as normal seasonal rises. According to the World Health Organization there has been no evidence so far of any widespread epidemic such as last year's Asian flu.[251]

This was actually one of the first times two nonlocal stories about the same country were framed differently. One had an alarmist tone and focused on fatalities, while the other acknowledged an epidemic, but neutralized, or confused, perceived fears.

Several days later, in another story by the *Times*'s correspondent, the headline read, "Flu Deaths Tripled in Britain in Week," and the story led off with "Influenza continued last week to be a serious peril to British health with the death rate rising more than threefold over the week before."[252] Further down in the story, the correspondent attributed a spokesman for the Ministry of Health as having said "influenza 'has now spread to many parts of the country'" and "in the great majority of cases the illness continues to be of a mild type, usually lasting only a few days."

Then the *New York Times* correspondent reported:

> The British Medical Association, however, had a different interpretation. A spokesman said that, although the influenza was of a mild variety, "it is taking considerably longer to get people back to work."[253]

This type of information was ambiguous and did not actually reappear for the duration of the British epidemic; it did maintain the frame that an epidemic was affecting many people.

A week later, it was reported that the flu epidemic in Britain had killed 1,125 Britons, and that

> [a] Ministry of Health spokesman said the flu this year appeared to have been even more severe than usual on old persons. Among last week's dead, 768 were 65 years old or older.
>
> The spokesman said the number of deaths was similar to that in the epidemic of 1953 and the Asian flu epidemic in 1957.[254]

This is actually the last story that ran in the *New York Times* about the British influenza epidemic. None of the stories reported whether England had changed its policy to mandate reporting influenza cases. Although a Ministry of Health spokesman was now willing to identify a high-risk group, there was no more mention of medical statistics.

Local coverage did, however, begin to chronicle outbreaks of influenza across the United States.[255] However, when outbreaks were reported, they were described as "mild" and to be "in normal limits."[256] In one local story the reason for alarm was explained by the New York City Bureau of Preventable Diseases Chief Dr. Morris Greenberg:

> Dr. Greenberg said the city had been watching particularly for influenza in view of reports of increased respiratory diseases and influenza this winter in Europe.[257]

The last several stories for 1959 did not actually discuss an influenza outbreak in the United States, but focused on remedies, such as a new live flu vaccine developed by a Russian scientist and in widespread use in the "Soviet Union."[258] Once the threat of Asian influenza had ended, so too did the coverage.

Coverage in *The Times* (London) after the pandemic up to December 1958 was sparse, focusing primarily on new research and scientific meetings.[259] It was reported that the 1957 Asian flu epidemic cost the national insurance program over ten million pounds sterling. On August 28, a story said:

> New outbreaks of Asian influenza are foreseen by the World Health Organization's expert committee on respiratory virus diseases. . . .
>
> The committee expect that the fresh outbreaks may prove milder because the natural resistance built up last year will make it more difficult for the virus to get about.[260]

In an editorial the next day, the framing of the Asian influenza virus up to this point was expressed literally. The editor said:

> At this time last year, as the new virus was sweeping irresistibly across the world, inevitable comparisons were made with the dread epidemic of 1918–1919. Fortunately, with that unpredictability which has always characterized influenza, the virus never assumed the virulent properties that were at one time feared.
>
> It is probable that the 1957–1958 epidemic was studied more carefully than any of its predecessors, and the experts who have been reviewing the prospects for the coming winter had therefore much information at their disposal when they met recently.[261]

The editorial attempted to relieve anxiety about the WHO's prediction of another influenza outbreak. It also reiterated the frame introduced during the Asian pandemic, which was fear of a repeat of the 1918 pandemic. Then the editorial illustrated how science had advanced and discussions about influenza viruses were more fluid, hence the WHO prediction.

The last *Times* (London) article for 1958 was a nonlocal story from Singapore, warning of Asian influenza. The article reported that a professor with the department of bacteriology at the University of Malaya said Asian influenza "was back in Singapore and Malaya, and could be expected to spread to Europe and Africa."[262] The article ended, saying, "A medical spokesman said, however, that the outbreak appeared to be on the wane and there was no cause for alarm." Regardless of the disclaimer, an alarm was raised and framed by the British press.

The first story for 1959 indexed for influenza in *The Times* (London) reported that nearly six hundred children had contracted a type of influenza similar to Asian influenza.[263] The article also said that this outbreak was a "very mild form."[264] On February 6, 1959, it was reported that schools were "badly hit by influenza."[265] The next day it was reported that "[d]octors in many districts of greater London are finding it hard to keep pace with influenza and other winter ailments."[266] About a week later, it was reported that

> there were 144 deaths from influenza in England and Wales in the week ended February 7, compared with 54 the previous week, figures issued by the General Register Office show. . . .
>
> The "red warning" for hospitals remains in force in the London area. The warning, sent out by the Emergency Bed Service, halts all but emergency admissions.[267]

The information framed by the press was that a serious epidemic was in England and it was affecting schoolchildren and the elderly. However, while deaths and infection rates were chronicled, the press continued to frame this influenza outbreak as "mild."[268] At the end of February, a long article was run about the cost of influenza to industry. The article recapped statistics about the 1957 Asian flu epidemic, but did not print any new information about the current epidemic. Due to the large losses to British businesses, the article said that a response was for some companies to initiate preventative measures to avoid the flu. While no new information was shed on the current epidemic in London, one could imply that the information presented was a general suggestion to those businesses fearful of their employees contracting the flu.

The next day, a story ran attributed to the Ministry of Health that said, "In most areas of Britain, however, reports show that the influenza peak is passing."[269] The articles that appeared over the next several months then detailed the decline of the epidemic. The last article indexed for 1959 in *The Times* (London) was a nonlocal story that said:

> About 70 passengers and members of the crew of the Union-Castle liner *Athlone Castle*, which docked at Southampton yesterday, were ill with influenza during a voyage from South Africa."[270]

There was no more mention of influenza, and like the stories in the *New York Times*, once the perceived threat had passed, so too did the indexed stories.

CONCLUSION

In addressing an overall theme for the social construction of disease for the 1957 Asian influenza pandemic, while the narrative discourse and implied health policies changed, the overall theme of cautious optimism did not.

The Asian flu pandemic of 1957 was dramatically different from the Spanish influenza pandemic in 1918 with regard to fatalities, but the magnitude of those infected and absent from schools and the workplace was dramatic, with up to 35 percent of the population afflicted. In searching for a way to frame the definition of the 1957 pandemic, many articles recalled the 1918 pandemic as a general reference point, which evoked a high level of public anxiety given the number of 1918 pandemic deaths. However, early on, the Asian pandemic was defined as a mild illness whose main public health issue was that of felling a population and disrupting essential services.

The narrative discourse raised by this pandemic was primarily of a theme of optimism and faith in science. News stories and editorials rallied to miracle drugs such as vaccines and antibiotics. While nonlocal coverage still tended along the lines of the previous pandemic, the alarmist narrative practically diminished and focused instead on either alerts, or following local coverage. The threat of an epidemic drove the amount of space devoted to debating how the local community would respond. Clearly, scientific advances were framed within the context of the fifties, and that was of a great trust and faith in new scientific advancements.

However, the very system that led this optimistic theme crashed when the vaccination supply could not meet the public's demand, especially in the United States, but then rallied to cautious optimism. New health policies ensued around the world in reference to just *who* would be considered a priority, given the insufficient supply. What resulted was a new frame in the public health philosophy, where consideration would eventually be given to those at medical risk, over a physician's preferential choice. The narrative frames about the very scientific advancements that were at the foundation for the theme of optimism were challenged. The effectiveness of a vaccine was debated. Antibiotic therapy was debated, and hospitalized care was also debated. While these debates were obvious frames carried in the American media coverage, in the British press they were undercurrents of overall frames of neutrality.

NOTES

1. "The Ghost of 1918: Influenza," *Today's Health* 34 (1956): 50–51.
2. Ibid.
3. Ibid.
4. "Influenza Epidemic in Bristol," *The Times*, 16 February 1956, p. 4.
5. "Telegrams in Brief," *The Times*, 9 March 1956, p. 8; "Influenza in Hull Trawler," *The Times*, 16 March 1956, p. 8; and "Influenza Epidemic," *The Times*, 19 March 1956, p. 8.
6. "60 Ill with Influenza at Bryanston School," *The Times*, 17 March 1956, p. 4.

7. B. Furman, "New Vaccine Aids in War on Grippe," *New York Times*, 17 August 1956, p. 21.
8. Ibid.
9. Ibid.
10. "130 Japanese Die of Influenza," *New York Times*, 14 December 1956, p. 10; and "130 Deaths in a Day From Influenza," *The Times*, 14 December 1956, p. 10.
11. "Flu: Another wave is overdue," *Changing Times* 11 (1957): 36.
12. "Influenza Besets Poland," *New York Times*, 20 March 1957, p. 4.
13. "Hong Kong Battling Influenza Epidemic," *New York Times*, 17 April 1957, p. 3.
14. Ibid.
15. "Taipei Fears Flu Epidemic," *New York Times*, 2 May 1957, p. 10.
16. "Britain Rushes Influenza Curb," *New York Times*, 7 June 1957, p. 12.
17. "350,000 Cases of Flu Reported by Bombay," *New York Times*, 4 June 1957, p. 3.
18. "London, June 5 (AP)," *New York Times*, 6 June 1957, p. 33.
19. "Influenza Epidemic Spreading In India," *New York Times*, 6 June 1957, p. 33
20. Ibid.
21. K. Love, "Britain Rushes Influenza Curb," *New York Times*, 7 June 1957.
22. Ibid.
23. B. Furman, "U. S. Acts To Bar Asian Influenza," *New York Times*, 8 June 1957, p. 22.
24. Ibid.
25. Ibid.
26. "Coast Cases Reported," *New York Times*, 8 June 1957, p. 22.
27. "Flu Vaccine Produced," *New York Times*, 9 June 1957, p. 22.
28. Ibid.
29. "Asian Influenza," *New York Times*, 9 June 1957, sec. 4, p. 10.
30. Ibid.
31. "Influenza Epidemic in Far East," *New York Times*, 9 June 1957, sec. 4 p. 11.
32. Ibid.
33. "Vaccine is Tested for Far East Flu," *New York Times*, 11 June 1957, p. 37.
34. "State Acts to Bar Far East Influenza," *New York Times*, 13 June 1957, p. 24.
35. Ibid.
36. Ibid.
37. "London, June 17," *New York Times*, 18 June 1957, p. 9; and "Flu Epidemic Linked to New Virus Type," *New York Times*, 19 June 1957, p. 16.
38. "Oriental Flu Tests On," *New York Times*, 20 June 1957, p. 60.
39. "Asian Flu Strikes East Coast Base," *New York Times*, 22 June 1957, p. 17.
40. Ibid.
41. "Asian Flu Epidemic," *New York Times*, 23 June 1957, p. 2.
42. Ibid.
43. "Flu Vaccine Produced," *New York Times*, 24 June 1957, p. 25.
44. "U.S. Acts to Combat Far East Influenza," *New York Times*, 26 June 1957, p. 9.
45. Ibid.
46. "Netherlands Acts Against Asian Flu," *New York Times*, 6 July 1957, p. 3.

47. "Influenza Vaccine," *New York Times*, 7 July 1957, sec. 4, p. 7.
48. Ibid.
49. "Tests Show Asian Flu," *New York Times*, 10 July 1957, p. 28.
50. Ibid.
51. "Vaccine Standards For Asian Flu Set," *New York Times*, 11 July 1957, p. 4.
52. "Asian Flu Hits 12,000," *New York Times*, 27 July 1957, p. 4.
53. Ibid.
54. Ibid.
55. Ibid.
56. "Asian Influenza," *New York Times*, 31 July 1957, p. 22.
57. Science Service, "Fertile Eggs Being Used For Asiatic Flu Vaccine," *New York Times*, 31 July 1957, p. 25.
58. Ibid.
59. B. Furman, "U.S. Flu Outbreak Called Probable," *New York Times*, 2 August 1957, p. 21.
60. Ibid.
61. "City Plans to Cope With Asiatic Flu; Committee Set Up," *New York Times*, 3 August 1957, p. 17.
62. "Flu Hits Labor Camps," *New York Times*, 7 August 1957, p. 16.
63. "Eisenhower Seeks Fund To Fight Flu," *New York Times*, 8 August 1957, p. 25.
64. Ibid.
65. Ibid.
66. "Asiatic Flu Cases Suspected in City, " *New York Times*, 9 August 1957, p. 21.
67. Ibid.
68. "8 Suspected Cases of Asian Flu Gain," *New York Times*, 10 August 1957, p. 33.
69. "Geneva, Aug. 9," *New York Times*, 10 August 1957, p. 33.
70. "Asiatic Flu Shots Start Next Month," *New York Times*, 11 August 1957, p. 46.
71. See "U.S. Flu Outbreak Called Probable," *New York Times*, 2 August 1957, p. 21; "Eisenhower Seeks Fund To Fight Flu," *New York Times*, 8 August 1957, p. 25; "Asiatic Flu Shots Start Next Month," *New York Times*, 11 August 1957, p. 46; and "Flu Affects 200 on Incoming Ship," *New York Times*, 13 August 1957, p. 29.
72. J. J. Ryan, "All But 27 Flu Cases on Liner Cleared for U.S. Travel," *New York Times*, 14 August 1957, p. 1.
73. F. Fowle, "Flu Offers Test Of City's Power," *New York Times*, 14 August 1957, p. 16.
74. Ibid.
75. Ibid.
76. "Student's Death is Linked to Flu," *New York Times*, 15 August 1957, p. 23.
77. L. Robinson," Flu Mapped by City and State," *New York Times*, 16 August 1957, p. 21; and "20,000 Hit By Flu in U.S. Since June," *New York Times*, 17 August 1957, p. 17.
78. R. K. Plumb, "Antibiotics and Vaccines are Prepared to Cope with Threat of Asiatic Influenza," *New York Times*, 18 August 1957, p. 9.
79. Ibid.
80. "Tigers, Big and Little," *New York Times*, 18 August 1957, sec. 4, p. 8.

81. B. Becker, "Harriman Urges 'Cop With A Billy,'" *New York Times*, 19 August 1957, p. 12.

82. Ibid.

83. "Vaccine For Flu Ordered By City," *New York Times*, 21 August 1957, p. 56.

84. "New Type of Influenza Officially Called Asian," *New York Times*, 24 August 1957, p. 33.

85. "Warning on Allergy," *New York Times*, 25 August 1957, p. 82.

86. W. L. Lawrence, "Eisenhower Gets an Asian Flu Shot," *New York Times*, 27 August 1957, p. 1.

87. Ibid.

88. "Flu Shot Priority Set for City Aids," *New York Times*, 28 August 1957, p. 25.

89. Ibid.

90. "More Flu Vaccine Made Available," *New York Times*, 29 August 1957, p. 29.

91. Ibid.

92. Ibid.

93. "Flu-Shot Life Set at 3 to 12 Months," *New York Times*, 29 August 1957, p. 29.

94. Ibid.

95. Ibid.

96. P. Kihss, "Flu Cases Urged to Rest at Home," *New York Times*, 31 August 1957, p. 17.

97. Ibid.

98. "Flu-Shot Life Set at 3 to 12 Months," *New York Times*, 29 August 1957, p. 29.

99. "Red Cross Urges Family Flu Fight," *New York Times*, 8 September 1957, p. 38.

100. "Odyssey of an Epidemic," *New York Times*, 1 September 1957, sec. 4, p. 8; and "Into the U.S. by Sea and Air," *New York Times*, 1 September 1957, sec. 4, p. 8.

101. "No Reason to Panic," *New York Times*, 1 September 1957, sec. 4, p. 8.

102. "Distributing Flu Vaccine," *New York Times*, 6 September 1957, p. 20.

103. R. K. Plumb, "Use of Antibiotics in Flu is Opposed," *New York Times*, 7 September 1957, p. 21.

104. Ibid.

105. "Red Cross Urges Family Flu Fight," *New York Times*, 8 September 1957, p. 38.

106. "Flu Discussion Here," *New York Times*, 8 September 1957, p. 38.

107. Ibid.

108. "State Priority List for Flu Shots Given," *New York Times*, 10 September 1957, p. 38.

109. *New York Times*, 10 September 1957, p. 38.

110. L. Robinson, "Flu Unit Declines to Ask Shots Now," *New York Times*, 11 September 1957, p. 35.

111. Ibid.

112. Ibid.

113. "State Unit Backs Flu Shots for All," *New York Times*, 13 September 1957, p. 44.

114. Ibid.

115. L. Robinson, "City Aide Predicts Big Flu Outbreak," *New York Times*, 14 September 1957, p. 20.

116. "Attitude Called Unrealistic," *New York Times*, 14 September 1957, p. 20.
117. "Suburbs Prepare for Threat of Flu," *New York Times*, 15 September 1957.
118. Ibid.
119. "2 British Crews Disabled By Flu," *New York Times*, 17 September 1957, p. 13
120. B. Furman, "Spread is Termed Rapid," *New York Times*, 17 September 1957, p. 13.
121. Ibid.
122. Ibid.
123. "No reason to Panic," *New York Times*, 4 September 1957, sec. 4, p. 8.
124. "Asian Flu," *New York Times*, 18 September 1957 p. 32.
125. "Firemen to Receive City's First Vaccine Against Flu Today," *New York Times*, 19 September 1957, p. 31.
126. "100,000 Flu Cases Reported in U. S." *New York Times*, 20 September 1957, p. 27.
127. "Allocation of Vaccine," *New York Times*, 25 September 1957, p. 31.
128. "Telegrams in Brief," *The Times*, 17 April 1957, p. 8.
129. "Far East Influenza Epidemic Spreading Towards Europe," *The Times*, 31 May 1957, p. 10.
130. Ibid.
131. Ibid.
132. "Spread Of Influenza in Asia," *The Times*, 5 June 1957, p. 9.
133. "Asian Influenza Precautions Taken," *The Times*, 6 June 1957, p. 4.
134. Ibid.
135. Ibid.
136. "Telegrams in Brief," *The Times*, 10 June 1957, p. 5.
137. "Flu Vaccine Produces," *New York Times*, 9 June 1957, p. 22.
138. "Influenza In Liner," *The Times*, 10 June 1957, p. 6.
139. "Combating 'Asiatic Influenza,'" *The Times*, 13 June 1957, p. 8.
140. Ibid.
141. "Influenza 'In Britain Next Winter,'" *The Times*, 17 June 1957, p. 10.
142. Ibid.
143. "Vaccine Against Asiatic 'Flu,'" *The Times*, 18 June 1957, p. 10.
144. Ibid.
145. "'Far East' Influenza Case Suspected," *The Times*, 18 June 1957, p. 10.
146. "Asian Influenza," *The Times*, 2 July 1957, p. 6.
147. Ibid.
148. "Four Arrivals with Asiatic Influenza." *The Times*, 9 July 1957, p. 13.
149. "MP Fears Early Flu Epidemic," *The Times*, 19 December 1968, p. 3.
150. "Preventing an Epidemic," *The Times*, 18 July 1957, p. 11.
151. Ibid.
152. "Virus from Asia," *The Times*, 23 July 1957, p. 9.
153. "Developing and Testing a Vaccine to Prevent Asian Flu," *The Times*, 29 July 1957, p. 16
154. "Influenza Pandemic," *The Times*, 31 July 1957, p. 9.
155. Ibid.
156. Ibid.

157. "Influenza Pandemic," *The Times*, 8 August 1957, p. 7.

158. "Influenza Test Successful," *The Times*, 9 August 1957, p. 3.

159. "'No Large Build-Up' at Present of Asian 'Flu in Britain," *The Times*, 31 August 1957, p. 4.

160. Ibid.

161. The word "seeded" used in this fashion can be traced back to narratives about the Black Death of 1348–1349.

162. "Britain 'Well Seeded With Asian Virus,'" *The Times*, 7 September 1957, p. 5.

163. "Vaccine Against Influenza," *The Times*, 12 September 1957, p. 10.

164. Ibid.

165. "Submarine Crews Have Influenza," *The Times*, 16 September 1957, p. 8.

166. "Biggest Western Exercise," *The Times*, 17 September 1957, p. 6; "Men In Sickbays," *The Times*, 17 September 1957, p. 6; and "'Atomic' Attacks in N.A.T.O. Exercise," *The Times*, 21 September 1957, p. 4.

167. "Influenza Still 'Mild,'" *The Times*, 23 September 1957, p. 4; and "12 Deaths in Week from Influenza," *The Times*, 24 September 1957, p. 5.

168. "Early Inoculation of Doctors," *The Times*, 23 September 1957, p. 4; and "'Flu Vaccine Distribution," *The Times*, 25 September 1957, p. 4.

169. P. Benjamin, "Asian Flu in City Called Epidemic; 150,000 Pupils Ill," *New York Times*, 3 October 1957, p. 1.

170. "Instructions on Care of Flu," *New York Times*, 1 October 1957, p. 3.

171. Ibid.

172. Ibid.

173. Ibid.

174. "Prince Charles Falls Ill," *New York Times*, 3 October 1957, p. 16.

175. "Queen Inoculated Against Asian Flu," *New York Times*, 10 October 1957, p. 5.

176. "70,000 Dutch Stricken Daily," *New York Times*, 3 October 1957, p. 16.

177. Ibid.

178. "Soviet Nationalizes Flu," New York Times, 13 October 1957, p. 65.

179. R. Alden, "Flu Cases Drop, Except in Queens," *New York Times*, 6 October 1957, p. 74; and R. Alden, "Flu Up in Schools; State Aid Imperiled," *New York Times*, 8 October 1957, p. 1.

180. L. Robinson, "Is It a Real Epidemic?" *New York Times*, 10 October 1957, p. 24.

181. Ibid.

182. Ibid.

183. Ibid.

184. P. Benjamin, "Physicians Score Flu Vaccine Lack," *New York Times*, 12 October 1957, p. 21.

185. Ibid.

186. F. Cohn, "Allocation of Flu Vaccine," *New York Times*, 14 October 1957, p. 26.

187. "Jailed in Flu Vaccine Theft," *New York Times*, 27 October 1957, p. 68.

188. "Flu Cases in U.S. Exceed 1,5000,000," *New York Times*, 18 October 1957, p. 25.

189. "Health Officials Optimistic on Flu," *New York Times*, 22 October 1957, p. 68.

190. B. Furman, "U.S. Predicts an Increase in Flu; Vaccine's Potency to be Doubled," *New York Times*, 24 October 1957, p. 1.

191. Ibid.

192. "Week's Flu and Pneumonia Toll is 2 1/2 Times Total in '56 Period," *New York Times*, 1 November 1957, p. 29.

193. "2D Flu Shot Urged with New Vaccine," *New York Times*, 3 November 1957, p. 50.

194. "Lethal Flu Epidemic Called New Threat," *New York Times*, 6 November 1957, p. 43.

195. Ibid.

196. Ibid.

197. "500,000 Here Hit by the Asian Flu," *New York Times*, 10 November 1957, p. 64.

198. R. K. Plumb, "Toll of Asian Flu Nothing Like 1918," *New York Times*, 15 November 1957, p. 29.

199. "National Decline in Flu Reported," *New York Times*, 22 November 1957, p. 52.

200. Ibid.

201. "Flu Severity Rises as New Cases Fall," *New York Times*, 6 December 1957, p. 31.

202. A. R. Hammer, "Vaccine in Surplus as the Flu Subsides," *New York Times*, 8 December 1957, sec. 3, p. 1.

203. "U.S. Finds Flu Put 50% in Nation in Bed," *New York Times*, 11 December 1957, p. 9.

204. Ibid.

205. "Asian Flu Wave Found Declining," *New York Times*, 13 December 1957, p. 41.

206. Ibid.

207. Ibid.

208. "U.S. Flu Deaths Rise," *New York Times*, 31 December 1957, p. 13.

209. "Rising Flu Deaths Spur U.S. Inquiry," *New York Times*, 8 February 1958, p. 21.

210. "2d Flu Wave Hits Milwaukee," *New York Times*, 12 February 1958, p. 16.

211. "Flu Shots Found Weak," *New York Times*, 15 February 1958, p. 19.

212. Ibid.

213. W. L. Lauwrence, "Influenza Strikes Again," *New York Times*, 16 February 1958, sec. 4, p. 9.

214. Ibid.

215. Ibid.

216. "Influenza Deaths Decline in a Week," *New York Times*, 15 March 1958, p. 19.

217. "City Deaths Rise in 2D Flu Wave," *New York Times*, 24 March 1957, p. 29.

218. "New Flu Variant is Studied by U.S.," *New York Times*, 25 March 1958, p. 30.

219. "Influenza Epidemic 'Underestimated,'" *The Times*, 17 October 1957, p. 10.

220. "Duke of Cornwall Has Influenza," *The Times*, 3 October 1957, p. 10; and "Vaccination for Queen," *The Times*, 10 October, 1957, p. 10.

221. See "Sharp Rise in Deaths from Influenza," *The Times*, 7 October 1957, p. 4; and "Influenza Deaths Up Slightly," 21 October 1957, p. 6.

222. "600 Influenza Deaths," *The Times*, 29 October 1957, p. 5.

223. Ibid.

224. "Fewer Deaths From Influenza," *The Times*, 4 November 1957, p. 5; "Further Decrease in Influenza Deaths," *The Times*, 11 November 1957, p. 4; "News in Brief," *The Times*, 18 November 1957, p. 6; and News in Brief," *The Times*, 25 November 1957, p. 6.

225. "Germs Resist Penicillin," *The Times*, 14 January 1958, p. 5.

226. Ibid.

227. Ibid.

228. "Toll of Influenza," *The Times*, 15 February 1958, p. 5.

229. Ibid.

230. "Upstate Flu Hit 850,000 Last Fall," *New York Times*, 1 April 1958, p. 33; and "Worse Flu Virus Suspected by City," *New York Times*, 31 May 1958, p. 17.

231. "Worse Flu Virus Suspected by City," *New York Times*, 31 May 1958, p. 17.

232. Ibid.

233. Ibid.

234. "Warns of Asian Flu," *New York Times*, 15 August 1958, p. 46.

235. Ibid.

236. "Influenza Shots Urged by U.S. Health Service," *New York Times*, 6 September 1958, p. 7.

237. Ibid.

238. "Asian Flu Downgraded as Threat This Winter," *New York Times*, 24 September 1958, p. 35.

239. Ibid.

240. "Asian Flu Recurs in Malaya," *New York Times*, 21 November 1958, p. 30.

241. "Flu Strikes Scout Jamboree," *New York Times*, 4 January 1959, p. 5.

242. Ibid.

243. "2 New Viruses Found; Cause Flu-Like Illness," *New York Times*, 7 February 1959, p. 39.

244. Ibid.

245. "Flu Rises in Britain; Prince Charles Ill," *New York Times*, 10 February 1959, p. 2.

246. "Burney in Warning on Outbreak of Flu," *New York Times*, 12 February 1959, p. 25.

247. Ibid.

248. Ibid.

249. "Flu Spreads in Britain," *New York Times*, 13 February 1959, p. 8.

250. "British Flu Toll Soars," *New York Times*, 15 February 1959, p. 13.

251. Ibid.

252. "Flu Deaths Tripled in Britain in Week," *New York Times*, 22 February 1959, p. 9.

253. Ibid.

254. "Flu Kills 1,125 Britons," *New York Times*, 1 March 1959, p. 34.

255. "Virus B Flu Reported," *New York Times*, 7 March 1959, p. 3.

256. "Influenza Identified," *New York Times*, 28 March 1959, p. 15.

257. P. Kihss "'Flurry' of Colds Reported Easing," *New York Times*, 9 April 1959, p. 33.

258. "M. Illson," Russians Develop Live Flu Vaccine," 21 October 1959, p. 45; and "Science Notes," *New York Times*, 25 October 1959, sec. 4, p. 9.

259. "British Tracing of Sputniks," *The Times*, 16 May 1958, p. 9; and "Protection Against Asian Influenza," *The Times*, 25 July 1958, p. 5.

260. "W.H.O. Forecasts Asian Influenza," *The Times*, 28 August 1958, p. 6.

261. "Influenza Outlook," *The Times*, 29 August 1958, p. 9.

262. "Warning on Asian Influenza," *The Times*, 16 December 1958, p. 7.

263. "News in Brief," *The Times*, 24 January 1959, p. 4.

264. Ibid.

265. "Schools Badly Hit by Influenza," *The Times*, 6 February 1959, p. 6.

266. "Influenza 'High in London,'" *The Times*, 7 February 1959, p. 6.

267. "Influenza Deaths Rise Sharply," *The Times*, 16 February 1959, p. 5.

268. "Rises in Influenza Cases," *The Times*, 20 February 1959, p. 7; and "More Influenza Deaths," *The Times*, 23 February 1959, p. 5.

269. "May Warmth in Many Areas," *The Times*, 28 February 1959, p. 6.

270. "News In Brief," *The Times*, 8 August 1959, p. 4.

THREE

INTRODUCTION

The 1960s represented a period of great scientific achievements and advancements for the world. The work begun in the 1950s regarding space exploration and organ transplantation was achieved during the 1960s. Man not only went into space in 1961 to circle the moon, but also landed and planted a flag on the moon's surface by the close of the decade. The attempts to transplant kidneys in the United States and France in 1950 from deceased people became ordinary surgical procedures with the ability to manipulate immunity, for which a Nobel award was given in 1960. The first heart transplant in South Africa by Christiaan Barnard occurred in 1967. The first successful heart transplant in Great Britain was in 1968, and the human genetic code was deciphered as well.

In reference to public health, several advancements were made, such as the development of an attenuated measles vaccine in 1963. The world's first successful blood transfusion was performed in New Zealand in 1963, revolutionizing trauma care and allowing for longer, more complicated surgical procedures. Hospice care was introduced in London for the terminally ill, and the battle with cancer was now a full-fledged war. The United States Public Health Service in Washington transferred the responsibility for tracking infectious diseases to the United States Communicable Disease Center (CDC) in Atlanta, Georgia, whose name eventually changed to the Centers for Disease Control and Prevention. Additionally, the philosophy of community responsibility for sanitation during the early twentieth century had now evolved to a philosophy of individual responsibility, with specialized medical services.

With all of the wonderful advancements and expanding services for individual health, disease did prove to be a continuous threat when, in 1969, the WHO had to admit that its plan to eradicate malaria had failed. Up to this point, no disease had actually been eradicated. They were just tamed with newer, more advanced vaccines.

BEFORE THE PANDEMIC: JANUARY 1967 THROUGH SEPTEMBER 1968

The first influenza story, January 7, 1967, was a nonlocal story in the *New York Times* about an influenza epidemic in the Soviet Union.[1] Over a month later, a report about a breach in medical secrecy on behalf of a Russian physician was reported. The article reported that a

> departure from tradition in an article in the British-American magazine *Lancet* in which a Soviet physician has reported current data on the influenza epidemic that has been sweeping much of the Soviet Union this year.[2]

The news value of the story was not that an epidemic was sweeping the Soviet Union, but that a Russian physician was sharing information. At this point, the Soviet Union was not a part of the WHO, and a code of silence existed between Soviet scientists and the rest of the world.

The next article to appear was in *Life* magazine, for the week February 10, 1967.[3] The magazine reported on a new antiviral drug that had just been approved by the Federal Drug Administration to be used to combat the A2 influenza strain. The drug, Symmetrel, was being prescribed in Italy, Thailand, Poland, and the U.S.S.R., in order to combat current epidemics of influenza. However, further down in the story, the magazine reported that "Symmetrel works no more effectively than a good Asian flu vaccine."[4] The debate upon the merits of this drug did resurface in newspaper coverage during the pandemic.

The next article to appear was in July 1967, and involved a prediction from Washington by U.S. Surgeon General William H. Stewart.[5] He forecasted an "outbreak of influenza next winter, especially in the East."[6] He then "urged that vaccine be used by those most seriously affected by epidemic flu, such as persons over 45 years old and individuals with chronic illnesses," and that immunization should begin as soon as "practicable" after October 1 and "ideally" be completed by early December.[7] The framing of this article established that a high-risk group was now firmly established with regard to public health policy, and that a specific age was defined for those at risk. It is important to note that during the 1960s, the average life expectancy was in the seventies, and that the retirement age had not been adjusted to what it is today.

The framing of a vaccine also changed with a call for people to be vaccinated before the start of the potential epidemic, instead of during the actual outbreak. The length of effectiveness for the vaccine, it appeared, was three to six months, and the epidemic was forecasted for the "late" winter months.[8] A new advisory committee was also referred to in the article, which was attributed for the vaccine information—The Public Health Service Advisory Committee on Immunization Practices.[9]

Later, on July 29, a story from the Cleveland Associated Press (AP), in the *New York Times*, reported that a group of volunteers were scheduled to "leave for Costa Rica next week to immunize virtually the entire country and help check the spread of disease throughout Central America."[10] This type of action demonstrated for the first time that vaccines were now used for a population other than the one that had manufactured it. This type of framing suggested that preventative measures were being taken to a global, rather than just a local level.

At the end of July 1967, articles chronicling new influenza research methodologies began to appear with some regularity. An article on July 29, 1967, said more effective methods were being used to manufacture vaccines needed for the upcoming epidemic.[11] Another research article at the beginning of October told of the connection between the influenza virus and animals.[12]

At the beginning of October a magazine article presented a general history of the 1918 and 1957 flu pandemics.[13] In a sidebar separate from the story, the magazine reiterated that public health authorities were calling for an epidemic during the "1967–1968 season." A week later, on October 8, a *New York Times* article reiterated the prediction for a harsh winter epidemic and that, "one reason for increased anxiety among public health officials this winter is the dormancy for several years of a form of Asian flu that first struck in 1957."[14] This was the second mention of the 1957 pandemic and the 1918 pandemic. Like the magazine article, the author of the newspaper article presented a history of the previous pandemics and updated current research.

On October 20, the CDC predicted that a major influenza epidemic would not be nationwide, but would be concentrated primarily in highly populated areas in the Northeast.[15] The framing of the article was similar to previous pandemic coverage, which was to put the public on alert and continue to urge inoculation. A prediction made by the CDC a year before the pandemic outbreak, however, was a first. Clearly, the previous pandemic coverage had an effect on when to activate the medical alert system regarding a new threat of a pandemic. These alerts, however, predicted an epidemic for January 1968, and were not focused on the entire 1968 flu season, October 1968 through March 1969.

On November 9, 1967, New York health officials said that there was "little likelihood of an Asian flu epidemic in New York this winter."[16] However, this position was reversed a week later and old frames emerged regarding the lack of enough vaccines for the entire population at the forefront of the coverage.[17] This time, New York City was also advocating a "high risk" priority group, but its definition was "those over 65, the chronically ill, and the institutionalized sick."[18] On November 26, while waiting for something to happen, another article presented a history of past influenza pandemics.[19]

The first signs that the anticipated epidemic had reached the United States, specifically in New York, were noted by the United States Public Health Service in Washington on December 21, 1967.[20] It was reported that this epidemic was a new strain of the A2 virus, and that persons "over 65 and those who already have chronic respiratory disease, heart disease or other conditions that weaken them seriously" be vaccinated. The article also reported:

> There is a difference of opinion among specialists on whether it does much good to take the vaccine in the midst of a local flu outbreak.
>
> Some say there is a reasonable probability that it may help. Others doubt it.
>
> "In areas where influenza activity is already known, it is probably too late," said Dr. Stephen Schoenbaum of the Respiratory Viral Disease Unit of the National Communicable Disease Center in Atlanta.[21]

The article also attributed doctors as having said that this epidemic was expected to be mild and did not show signs of severe or unusual numbers of fatalities. However, another story, also attributed to the CDC, reported that deaths were already higher than usual.[22] A couple of days later, a nonlocal story reported that the epidemic was also present in London.[23]

Through mid-January, stories in the *New York Times* chronicled the infection rates and fatalities in New York, as well as the rest of the United States, and that the epidemic was now labeled the Asian flu.[24] Officials maintained that this epidemic was "primarily of the A-2 strain which runs a relatively mild, self-limited course in average adults."[25] By January 10, 1968, health officials said that the New York City flu epidemic had reached a severe stage, but that it was "expected to abate after the next week."[26] A January 12 editorial reiterated current scientific knowledge of influenza and that "the present spasm of cases seems to fall in the class of relatively mild epidemics."[27]

In the Sunday paper, a couple of days later, a profile by Jane Brody presented a narrative about how the flu was affecting office managers.[28] Two days later, another article said that the "influenza epidemic that has plagued New Yorkers for five weeks has reached its peak and is expected to decline."[29]

It is notable that in the initial coverage for this epidemic, there was no information of a vaccine shortage, and that the theme was optimistic, with a warning only to the high-risk population. The style of writing was not hard news, punctuated by public health mishaps or shortcomings, as compared to the previous pandemics. Previously, this type of coverage emerged at the end of the Asian flu pandemic and only after the epidemic had passed. There were also more bylined local news stories of the epidemic rather than by correspondents out of Washington.

While the epidemic passed through the United States, the first mention of an actual decline in death rates appeared on January 23, 1968.[30] All of the articles used statistical information as evidence and explained how the CDC tracked the figures both locally and nationally.[31] By February 3, the CDC reported that the flu death rate had declined for most of the United States.[32] The coverage then switched back to discussing a new type of flu vaccine and nonlocal reports of influenza.[33]

A couple of months later, on April 15, the *New York Times* reported that the Fiji islands had been struck by a severe epidemic of influenza.[34] On July 7, 1968, the CDC then reported that it "did not expect any widespread outbreaks of influenza during the winter of 1968–1969 in the United States."[35] On September 1, 1968, "The Health Department in Manila placed the entire Philippines under an influenza alert," said a nonlocal Reuters story.[36]

On September 5, the CDC reversed its earlier prediction. The article in its entirety said:

> The Public Health Service Advisory Committee predicted today that a new strain of Asian flu might cause an extensive outbreak in the United States this fall and winter.
>
> The committee, which had forecast the opposite in July, revised its prediction because of the appearance of a new strain in Hong Kong.
>
> The earlier prediction was made because the country experienced a rather wide-spread incidence of Asian flu last year and it was expected that a natural immunity would provide protection.
>
> However, the committee said that the new strain from Hong Kong showed marked antigenic changes from previous strains and that there was no specific vaccine available for the strain called "A2-Hong Kong-68."[37]

The information in this story quite literally emphasized the potential for a true emergency. There was no debate about a prediction mistake, as the article addressed why the mistake happened. This was also the first mention of an official name for the virus, which would later become known as the Hong Kong pandemic of 1968.

On September 17, a couple of weeks before the flu season, an article written by Jane E. Brody said:

> Manufacturers are working full speed to produce a vaccine for a new virus strain that threatens to cause an influenza epidemic in this country this winter.
>
> Unfortunately, the vaccine manufacturers can work only as fast as the new virus will grow in the laboratory, and how fast that will be, no one yet knows.
>
> Estimates of when an effective vaccine will be ready range from three to six months. Even then, enough vaccine probably will not be available in time to protect all those who are likely to be hardest hit by influenza—the chronically ill and elderly.[38]

This was the first time that a potential problem with a vaccine shortage was brought up by the press, unlike the reactionary reporting that occurred during the previous pandemics. This is also the first time in any pandemic coverage where the reason for the problem (vaccine shortage) was not blamed on public health officials, manufacturers, or unfair priority lists. Instead, the blame for the vaccine shortage was placed on nature. While previous coverage of influenza had hinted that the virus was naturally occurring, none expressed this frame as literally as this article did.

Further down in the story, Brody explained that the vaccines being distributed to doctors at the present time are "expected to provide only limited protection against the new virus."[39] She also explained why the epidemic was named A2-Hong Kong-68:

> The new strain is a variant of the A2 flu virus, which caused a worldwide epidemic in 1957. It is officially named A2/Hong Kong/68 because it first showed up in July in Hong Kong during an outbreak that left about 25 dead.[40]

She added that "influenza experts" said that the Hong Kong strain "causes a relatively mild illness about as severe as that caused by the old A2 virus."[41] The high-risk priority parameters were reiterated at the end of the article in reference to who should be vaccinated first with the new vaccine.

Approximately two weeks after the prediction of the Hong Kong epidemic, and ten days after the Brody article, another article by Brody with a headline read: "9 Cases of New Asian Flu are Reported in U.S."[42] Brody led off with:

> Hong Kong flu is here in the United States.
>
> The National Communicable Disease Center in Atlanta announced yesterday that it has received reports of nine cases of Hong Kong flu among United States residents. A spokesman for the center said there had doubtless been more like them that had not been reported.
>
> The illness, caused by a new strain of influenza virus called A2-Hong Kong-68, has been occurring in widespread outbreaks in the Far East since June.
>
> Two of the United States cases were an Atlanta businessman and his wife, who had contracted the virus on a trip to the Far East.[43]

This article was very straightforward, and framed the epidemic as a potential threat that was spread from the Far East. However, information in reference to the epidemic was updated from a start date of July 1968 to June 1968. The article reiterated the manufacturing process for a new vaccine, its shortfalls, and that the disease was expected to be mild, with "a four or five-day illness accompanied by malaise, fever, cough, headache and muscle ache."[44] What was not known was to what extent the public would be infected. The article ended with a scientist who said that "so far, it hasn't been growing too well," in reference to the manufacture of a suitable vaccine. From this one could infer that there might be an additional delay in the availability of a new vaccine.

Coverage by *The Times* (London) prior to the pandemic began on January 16, 1967, with a nonlocal story.[45] The very small article simply said, "An influenza wave is sweeping Poland. More than 15,000 people have already been affected."[46] Four days later, a story ran from Geneva and said:

> The appearance, perhaps in two or three years, of a completely new strain of influenza is predicted by the World Health Organization. This will emerge from the Asian influenza virus A2, first identified in 1957, which says W.H.O., is still very widespread, but is undergoing change. W.H.O. now has 76 influenza centres covering 53 countries. Their work is coordinated by the world influenza centre in London.[47]

This story did not run in the *New York Times*, nor was it attributed in any of the influenza stories for the same time period. *The Times* (London) article framed the possibility of a new threat and a "completely new strain of influenza," which would require a new vaccine. The next day another very short story said that more than 62,000 people in Warsaw had been affected by an influenza epidemic.[48] Another short story, some four months later, reported that a doctor at the World Influenza Centre in London said "that there was no sign of the world influenza outbreak expected by some experts to occur this year."[49]

However, at the end of December 1967, nearly seven months later, an influenza epidemic was reported in a local story, and that influenza had "attacked hundreds of people in London and southern England during the Christmas holiday."[50] This was the first page-one story to appear in *The Times* (London), but as previously noted, this was the first year in this study that *The Times* used page one for news information, rather than classified information. The story said, "Extra doctors were called in at the Emergency Call Service to deal with the severity of the attack but it was emphasized that there was no cause for alarm."[51]

The article framed the epidemic as mild, but sudden. Next to the influenza article on page one, was another story about a highly infectious "gastro-enteritis" epidemic that had already killed ten babies. According to the article, the infection originated in hospitals. This type of story, next to one about influenza called a past frame to mind, for which hospitals in Great Britain were blamed for staphylococcus infections that increased the death rates during the 1957 pandemic. While the actual influenza article was not very alarmist, the context in which it was placed and presented was.

The next day another page-one story about the influenza epidemic emphasized an alarmist frame and said:

> London hospitals yesterday received a "red alert" from the London Emergency Bed Service warning them to admit only patients needing urgent treatment.
>
> The alert was issued because of extra calls from doctors seeking hospital beds particularly from people with pneumonia and bronchitis. It follows the spread of influenza in London and other parts of Britain.[52]

The article also explained that the virus was not new and would probably subside in a week. Next to this story was another story explaining that the babies who had died did not die from a hospital-induced infection, thus lessening the severity of the potentially perceived threat of the day before. However, the next day, December 29, a page-one story headline read: "'Flu' Virus Kills Five Babies."[53] The story said that the virus that killed the babies had not been identified, but the headline, contextually, was framed otherwise. The body of the story reported that "the virus was not a hospital infection and the children who had died in hospital were all very ill when they were admitted."[54] The article also incorporated the phrase "chest illnesses" to refer to those stricken with influenza. Information in this article produced a narrative that reflected an alarmist reaction to the current influenza epidemic in Great Britain, which used contradictory information similar to the reporting during the first pandemic.

Another story in the business section of the paper detailed how the flu epidemic had boosted the British economy. Those positively affected by the epidemic were drug manufacturers, druggists, and "paper handkerchief makers."[55] This was the first story of an economic profit made during a pandemic for any of the media coverage.

The next day a second-page headline described the deaths of two more babies. While the headline clearly read, "'Flu epidemic kills two babies," the body of the story did not contain any such information, but instead said that the "coroner is waiting for the result of the post-mortem examinations which may be released today."[56] This type of coverage for *The Times* (London) was a complete departure from previous pandemic and epidemic coverage of the past. It seemed with the addition of a front page for which to attract readers, *The Times* had also begun to use contextual framing devices, such as alarmist headlines, to attract further attention and to attenuate the epidemic situation in London.

In the same newspaper, on page four, a story by the "Nature-Times News Service," presented another history of the influenza virus.[57] The information was factual and reiterated previous information about the different strains of an influenza virus. It said:

> Although the influenza outbreak, which is thought to have started in London and Liverpool, seems to be spreading, there is no suggestion yet that a major epidemic is imminent. The virus responsible—identified as type A2—is, in fact, very similar to, but not identical with, that which caused the world-wide Asian influenza pandemic in 1957.[58]

Several days later a story related that the red alert system for hospitals would continue, and that influenza-related fatalities from the week of December 22 were 101 for England and Wales.[59] The epidemic was framed as severe, with no predictions regarding its peak or abatement given. The next day a page-one story reported that the demand for hospital beds "soars," and that one hospital was turning away patients because "nearly 70 nurses have influenza."[60]

On January 4, a page-two story reported that "the influenza epidemic has affected London's postal services and the Post Office said yesterday that there would be delays to deliveries."[61] It is interesting to note that this story appeared under the section "In Brief," and that the only information from the Ministry of Health was fatality statistics. There was no mention of a vaccine of any kind. The framing suggested a relationship to the severity of the epidemic, with no preventative information given by *The Times*, which is a complete departure from previous coverage.

The next day, the severity of the epidemic continued to be framed with a page-two story that said:

> A waiting room at one of Brighton's hospitals has been turned into a temporary mortuary and one cemetery has brought in a mechanical digger to make graves after a sharp increase in the town's death rate over the past 10 days. About 300 people have died during the cold spell and influenza epidemic.[62]

The framing of this story was very alarmist and did nothing to calm public anxiety. On January 6 in a page-three story a headline read, "Influenza Deaths 101 in Week," and the story detailed the ravages of the epidemic across England.[63] At the end of the story was a report of the progress of the epidemic in the United States for the same time. It said that New York City was the hardest hit and that "reports from 122 cities in the United states showed that 613 persons died of pneumonia or flu during the week ending December 30." The "Staff Reporter" attributed information about the United States from the CDC. The coverage up to this point was probably the most severe of any reported in this study. The framing of intense suffering with no balance for preventative measures was remarkable. Absent, too, were any reports as to how the royal family was fairing with the flu epidemic.

Then, on January 10, 1968, as suddenly as the reports announced a deadly epidemic in London, another article reported that there was a decrease in hospital admissions.[64] One last story in reference to this epidemic reported that there had been a "fall in the mechanical and electrical industries' index" during the last quarter of 1967, which was probably attributable to the flu.[65] The next story indexed for influenza was not until six months later, on July 30, 1968, which reported a new strain of the Asian flu in Hong Kong in the science section of *The Times*. The article said:

> The "mild" epidemic of Asian influenza which has incapacitated about 400,000 people in Hong Kong and neighbouring areas in China could conceivably spread to Britain. The virus responsible is almost certainly of the same sub-type—A2—as the one that swept the world in 1957 and which has been responsible for several outbreaks since then, including the outbreak in London and Liverpool last December.[66]

The last sentence in the article said, "Whatever path the virus takes, the supplies of vaccine in Britain, which contain type A and B virus strains, should be sufficient to protect everyone without natural immunity." The framing of this story was not alarmist and the public was even told not to worry, since Great Britain has enough vaccines for everyone. This framing was calm with preventative measures guaranteed to the British public.

On August 9 a *Times* (London) article said a "wave of influenza" had struck Australia, and that the Australian premier, David Brand, had to halt the Legislative Assembly for a week.[67] Then, a month later, on September 10, the coverage switched to chronicling a race for Great Britain to develop a suitable vaccine for a new strain of influenza, A2, Hong Kong 1 /68.[68] (This frame reflected the framing of the Hong Kong epidemic by the *New York Times*.) It was now feared, *The Times* (London) reported, that this new influenza virus would be "an extensive epidemic."[69]

PANDEMIC COVERAGE: OCTOBER 1968 THROUGH MARCH 1969

Initial coverage during the flu season in the *New York Times* turned to the matter at hand, which was producing a vaccine that could protect Americans from the anticipated flu.[70] While manufacturers were attempting to grow a suitable vaccine culture, an article appeared in reference to a drug reported by *Life* magazine the previous year.[71] It turned out that the drug company, having received FDA approval for the use of the drug with the A2 influenza strain, did some preliminary testing against the new Hong

Kong strain and found the drug to have some effectiveness in animals. However, the company did not test the drug on humans and had to withdraw advertisements stating effectiveness against the new influenza strain until the drug had been properly tested.

Nonlocal coverage in the *New York Times* reiterated previous influenza framing devices by reporting on the severity of influenza elsewhere. On November 2, 1968, an article released from Geneva by the WHO said that the Hong Kong flu "has spread rapidly but had caused very few deaths since it had first been identified in Hong Kong last July."[72] The next day, an AP story from Rome reported that "200,000 persons are ill with 'Mao Tse-tung flu' in Rome alone."[73] The article explained the new "nickname," saying "the influenza virus got its nickname because it is believed to have originated in China and to have spread through Asia toward Europe via Hong Kong."[74] This type of coverage emphasized the old frame to place blame for the virus on a foreign country.

Additionally, for this pandemic, it appeared that research to produce a new vaccine was occurring in multiple labs across the country, with the race to produce a vaccine no longer framed as an international one. Now labs within the United States were racing amongst each other to produce the first batch of usable vaccines. One article said up to "seven pharmaceutical companies in the United States are producing a vaccine."[75]

By mid-November, the CDC reported that a "vaccine against the new strain of Asian flu will be available by the end of November."[76] The article also reiterated that "the chronically ill and elderly will be the first" to be vaccinated. Information from this story was reiterated in a local story for New York City.[77] However, the New York article included some new information. According to the pharmaceutical association, the article said, "'substantial quantities'" of vaccines would be available sometime after January 1, and that the majority of the early doses available would go to the military. This type of priority distribution was used during the Asian flu pandemic. However, this was the first mention of inoculating the military before high-risk civilians. The article ended with the reiteration that the Public Health Service "has recommended that the vaccine be given only to persons over age 65 and chronically ill."[78] The narrative in this article set up the potential for another debate about who would be vaccinated, with conflicting information from the United States Public Health Service and the pharmaceutical association, who were overseeing the production and distribution of the vaccine. However, if there was a problem, it was not actually stated in this article.

On November 20, the *New York Times* ran a story that said:

> The first Government-approved batch of Hong Kong influenza vaccine began the trip today to hospitals, pharmacies and doctors' offices across America. Officials are hopeful of checking a possible Asian flu epidemic.[79]

Right after this article was another from Washington that said:

> The Surgeon General of the United States Public Health Service asked doctors yesterday to reserve Hong Kong flu vaccine for "high risk" patients who might die without it.
>
> "If this follows the usual pattern, we should have a few outbreaks from now through December and then in January have a real epidemic," Dr. William H. Stewart said in an interview.[80]

This type of reportage inferred that the prioritizing of who should be vaccinated followed a "recommended" prioritizing of inoculation and was dependent upon the local physician's judgment. While this could be considered a public health policy, it was a voluntary one, unlike the previous pandemic where local jurisdictions decided priority list policies. The second article also included a prediction from the surgeon general as to when the epidemic was expected to hit hardest. All of the information was presented objectively, with the responsibility for vaccination left up to physicians on a case-by-case basis. Coverage then turned to chronicling outbreaks across the United States.[81] The first deaths reported were five residents at "the city's home for the aged" in Philadelphia.[82]

On December 4, 1968, an article from Houston reported:

> Apollo 8 astronauts received injections and started a program of "limited exposure" this week in a plan that doctors hope will keep them free of colds or influenza during their Christmastime flight around the moon.[83]

The article also said that

> back-up and support crews for Apollo 8, scheduled for launching Dec. 21, also received the shots, as did the prime, back-up and support crews of Apollo 9, scheduled for launching in February.[84]

Prior to this article, the only people singled out for news coverage about receiving flu vaccines were high-ranked politicians and the British royal family. The narrative of this particular article framed the country's focus on new space technology by covering the astronauts. Likewise, the article illustrated that the potential flu epidemic was also at the forefront of the American consciousness.

On December 5, 1968, a local article by Jane E. Brody detailed influenza outbreaks in New York City and said:

> If you are feeling achy, feverish and miserable without the will or the way to do much of anything, chances are you have the Hong Kong flu.
>
> The flu, which was virtually absent from the city last week descended upon an unknown number of unsuspecting New Yorkers starting Monday,

knocking out of commission the shipping departments of some concerns, the mail rooms of others.

Dr. Vincent Guinée of the city health department calls them "small outbreaks scattered widely all over the city, usually affecting groups of people who work together but not yet causing unusually high absenteeism in industry."

"This is just the beginning; the worst is yet to come," was Dr. Guinée's ominous prediction.[85]

This type of reportage was the first that took on a truly alarmist tone of what was actually expected by public health officials. Up to this point, officials had concerned themselves with identifying the epidemic and the production of a vaccine. The article also explained that school absenteeism would be difficult to ascertain because students in New York City were striking and already absent. Brody detailed other areas that were affected by the flu, such as theaters and other businesses. Near the end of the story, a new influenza frame emerged that gave, for the first time, detailed information about the transfer of the virus.

Influenza is most communicable during the first three days after the start of symptoms. Its incubation period is 24 to 72 hours, so if you were exposed Sunday and have not gotten sick yet, you won't—at least, not as a result of that contact.[86]

The article ended with a reiteration of high-risk persons to be inoculated before the general public, and that the vaccine was due in about two weeks. The framing of this influenza epidemic was that it was mild, a nuisance, and "is no better nor worse than last year's flu."[87]

By December 13, 1968, a report from the CDC said that the Hong Kong flu had now reached epidemic levels across the United States.[88] The article said:

Deaths from pneumonia and influenza have exceeded normal expectations, and the nation is in the midst of an epidemic of Hong Kong flu, the National Communicable Disease Center reported today.[89]

The article also said that the latest national death statistics demonstrated an increase in deaths across the United States. The narrative theme for the Hong Kong influenza epidemic in the United States was now framed in a truly alarmist fashion with deaths exceeding public health officials' expectations. The article then chronicled individual outbreaks across the United States, with an emphasis on the negative side effects of the epidemic on businesses, schools, and lives.

The next day, the Hong Kong flu epidemic was on page one in the *New York Times*. The story said that

[t]he Hong Kong flu, spreading at an ever faster rate, led yesterday to restrictions on hospital visitors here, the closing of colleges throughout the

> country, a slowdown in the nation's business and industrial activity and a threat to Christmas mail deliveries.
>
> National and local health authorities agreed that the worst was still to come, with the peak not expected until about the middle of next month. They hoped the highly infectious disease would taper off in February.[90]

This article also reflected a very alarmist tone regarding the epidemic and described the actual impact. A prediction was given for the proverbial light at the end of the tunnel, that it was hoped the epidemic would taper off in February and that vaccines should be available in one week. The effect of the epidemic on health policy is evidenced by the lead, with most of the policies unforeseen and voluntary.

The same day, an editorial ran that attempted to explain the virus by using a chameleon analogy. It said, "It changes chemical nature from year to year, returning in altered form each time to pose a new menace to its victims."[91] This type of information was a return to the frame that influenza was an act of nature that had not succumbed to man's scientific endeavors.

The next day Hong Kong officials challenged the name of the epidemic. The Hong Kong doctors "denounced foreign newspapers and foreign health authorities for tagging it with the colony's name."[92] They claimed that the flu actually originated in China and should be given "its proper name—China flu."[93] The framing device in this article was a literal reaction to the tendency for health officials to want to name influenza epidemics with a name other than their own. The article emphasized the signifying context of naming an influenza epidemic as a negative rhetorical framing device. Therefore, the article literally explained that blame was assigned when a virus was given a name.

On December 17, a letter to the editor illustrated the public's reaction to the vaccine frame:[94]

> The Times report (Dec. 11) that only five million doses of vaccine against the Hong Kong virus had been approved for distribution is disturbing.
>
> We are, we keep telling ourselves, a computerized and highly technological society whose blessing (or curse) is think-tank pre-analysis combined with push button control.
>
> Surely there has been a breakdown in both Governmental direction and free enterprise planning if we are left so unprotected, so late through the danger period, especially when the vaccine formula per se was in existence.
>
> This appears to be still another example of how our affluent society seems to get rather poor value for its proliferate dollars.[95]

The letter suggested that given the timing of information as reported by the media, a vaccine should have been made available in time to combat the epidemic. It was interesting to note that the time period for the influenza epidemic was now a common socially constructed notion.

The spread of the flu continued to be chronicled, with an emphasis on societal effects, an infection rate of 20 percent, and that the disease was still relatively mild.[96] A link was also drawn between the 1957 pandemic and the current epidemic by New York City Health Commissioner Dr. Edward O'Rouke who said that the infection rate of 25 percent "was as severe as the worldwide Asian flu epidemic of 1957."[97] Toward the end of the article, a couple of extra symptoms were added to the flu epidemic such as "a lack of will to do anything, and many victims report an inability to concentrate on simple tasks." And, although there was no medication the could halt the disease, one business, Edward Gottlieb and Associates, was reported to be giving its employees each afternoon a glass of orange juice mixed with cognac. The company claimed that it had had very little absenteeism, but it was also reported that the company "represents French cognac producers in the United States."[98] This type of framing was consistent with previous frames already established during the 1957 pandemic. However, the cognac incident, while reminiscent of the 1918 pandemic, was not reiterated during the 1957 pandemic, and was questionable given the self-serving interests of the business interviewed.

The next day, another *New York Times* article reported that 80,000 vaccines were given to "health centers, hospitals, nursing homes and homes for the aged that have requested it."[99] The priority of inoculating high-risk patients was again reiterated in a more direct fashion by the city health commissioner, who said, "Priority in administering the vaccine will be given to persons aged 65 and over and persons with chronic heart and respiratory diseases."[100] The article also reported that the American Red Cross had issued a directive "labeling the flu epidemic a 'disaster situation.'"[101] This type of coverage did not imply that the epidemic was just framed in an alarmist fashion, but described literally that the epidemic was a societal disaster.

The next day, December 19, 1968, a front-page story with a large photo and headline said, "City Attacks Flu As 200 Get Shots."[102] The photo was of a doctor giving an injection to an elderly man, with several other elders lined up for their vaccines at a New York City Board of Health Clinic. The story framed New York City as the responsible party that was taking control of the current epidemic situation. The author of the article used fight rhetoric to further illustrate the battle the city was involved in with influenza. In the body of the story he said:

> The first blow here to arrest the epidemic was struck in a Board of Health clinic, where 200 people received injections of the new vaccine calculated to prevent the ailment, which sometimes develops into pneumonia.[103]

The vaccines were also referred to as "preventative injections," which was the first time that the vaccine had been framed this way. Further down in the story, it was noted that President Johnson was in the hospital "with a bad cold and a fever." This reiterated the frame that officials were not taking the epidemic lightly.

The same day an editorial said:

> Judged by every criterion except loss of life, the current influenza epidemic is already one of the worst in the nation's history. There is no way of totaling the amount of discomfort and distress suffered by the millions who have already been hit. It is evident that the economic cost of this medical disaster—the amount spent for treating victims plus the associated loss of production from those who have had to go to bed instead of work—will amount to billions of dollars. In Hong Kong, one of every five persons contracted the ailment; if the same ratio holds true here this country will have had forty million flu patients before the ordeal ends.
>
> Is this huge human and economic cost necessary? The question arises inevitably now that the first grossly inadequate amounts of Hong Kong flu vaccine are beginning to become available.[104]

The editor essentially reiterated the severity of this epidemic and then questioned if it could have been avoided. He answered his question by saying that while nature does not allow for one to know exact information about when an epidemic will strike, this epidemic could have been "mounted," "if full advantage had been taken of existing knowledge."[105] But, the editor pointed out, "such a full-scale defense effort would cost much more than is normally spent on the preparation of vaccines."[106] The editor concluded:

> Congress and the public health agencies would do well to take another look at this aspect of the nation's medical protective system and to determine whether a Federally financed program unhampered by normal commercial factors, would not be a sound investment to prevent future epidemics.[107]

As the flu epidemic spread, two new issues developed and were incorporated into the flu coverage. First, a fuel shortage was said to complicate matters, and then a blood shortage was noted.[108] The fuel shortage was noted on December 20 in an article that said:

> Flu victims who are also forced to combat the cold may be more likely to suffer complications as a result of their illness, Dr. Edward O'Rourke, city Health Commissioner, said yesterday.
>
> The Commissioner made the comment to explain yesterday's declaration by the Board of Health that the city was in a 'state of imminent peril to pub-

> lic health' as a result of the fuel drivers' strike concurrent with the outbreak of Hong Kong flu.[109]

Whether this was a political ploy to end a strike is of no consequence. That another burden was framed within the influenza epidemic narrative was. In between this story and the next in reference to the fuel shortage and flu, were several stories that continued to frame this influenza epidemic as severe and ongoing.[110] One article reported that the first cases of Hong Kong flu in Britain were detected.[111] Another said "one of the sectors hit hard by the flu epidemic has been the executive branch of Government."[112]

Christmas day, a front-page story in the *New York Times* led off with:

> A shortage of heat, vaccine and blood plagued the city yesterday as the Hong Kong flu epidemic continued, and the Health Commissioner warned that many sick people might die unless emergency fuel deliveries were made.[113]

Now, not only was the city in the midst of an influenza epidemic, it was "plagued" by the lack of fuel, blood, and enough vaccines. According to the story, the vaccines had run out the day before, and "a critical shortage of blood was reported by the Greater New York Blood Program."[114] The fuel shortage due to the strike had been resolved, but the backlog of deliveries had not, the article explained.

Over the next week, the fuel shortage gained a considerable amount of attention while fuel companies attempted to catch up.[115] In a page-one story on December 28, it was reported that all the New York City schools would close for two days because of the lack of fuel.[116] The situation was dubbed "the fuel and flu crises."[117] However, by December 29, the fuel crisis in New York City was reported to have abated, while the blood shortage increased and the flu continued to spread.[118] The health commissioner said, "The flu epidemic, which has cut the number of blood donors and attendants in blood centers, is continuing unabated," and further explained the framing of the blood shortage with the flu epidemic.[119]

Daily coverage through to the first week of 1969 chronicled the effect the flu had on the blood shortage, which affected elective surgeries, which then exacerbated trauma surgeries.[120] The framing of influenza was now a socially constructed catastrophe, despite the fact that deaths did not account for the mayhem. However, on January 1, 1969, the *New York Times* did report that the flu epidemic had begun to abate:[121]

> The Hong Kong flu epidemic, while abating, is by no means over, Commissioner O'Rourke warned yesterday. He estimated that 600,000 to 700,000 more people would be afflicted with it before the epidemic ended. The number of cases so far is 900,000, he said.[122]

The announcement was very cautious, but steadied the heightened frame of alarm.

While the fuel and blood shortages were being dealt with, the vaccine shortage was also abated. For every article that mentioned the blood supply or the fuel supply, a sentence would notify the public that vaccines were being shipped and distributed on almost a daily basis. One article explained that "anyone between 21 and 64 who had not had flu for at least a week" could donate blood.[123] It was also significant to note that while this expanded framing of the influenza epidemic was being covered by the *New York Times*, there were very few words devoted to the national and international influenza epidemic.

On January 3, the New York City flu epidemic was reported to have "peaked earlier this week, and has continued to decline since" and that New York City was still in a "state of peril."[124] Right next to the epidemic article was another medical story that said that the first heart transplant patient of the year was recovering in "almost excellent condition" at a local New York City hospital.[125] Contextually, one could infer that the epidemic was receiving as much attention as two very popular topics for this time period—Astronauts in space and organ transplantation.

The next day the CDC reported that flu deaths had totaled 3,594 in four weeks in 122 cities across the United States.[126] However, the CDC also reported that the epidemic was beginning to subside nationwide. While the flu was easing up in New York, health officials continued to bring in vaccines to inoculate the general public. The article also reported that blood donations were up and reiterated the criteria for donation for anyone who had fallen ill with the flu. The shortage of fuel and its effects on the city's flu victims was also reiterated.[127] Therefore, the expanded frame of influenza with the blood and fuel shortage continued to be incorporated into one story, maintaining the frame begun at the onset of the three crises.

A day later, a United Press International (UPI) story from London reported that influenza deaths had "increased by nearly nine times in 1968," and that "a total of 4,311 persons in Britain died of flu last year."[128] On January 7, 1969, New York City ended its "state of imminent peril," which the article said had been brought on by the "combination of Hong Kong flu and the fuel oil strike."[129] The blood shortage was mentioned at the end of the article as having "balanced" out.

Three days later, a story from Geneva said:

> Outbreaks of the Hong Kong flu are now being reported from various European countries for the first time, the World Health Organization said today.
>
> In West Germany 17 cases developed at the end of December in a unit of the United States Army that included soldiers who had just returned from the United States.[130]

This time, the framing of the spread of an influenza epidemic was from the United States to Europe. Further down in this story it was reported that the Hong Kong flu epidemic was

> on its way to the Soviet Union and the nation is preparing to meet it. Tass, the Soviet press agency, said that large-scale vaccination was under way.[131]

Another story below said that "3,079 deaths could be attributed to the Hong Kong flu" in the United States.[132] As the flu declined in the United States, along with local coverage, nonlocal stories increased, which had been the case for each pandemic. Several articles continued to report on the spread of the Hong Kong flu in London, the Soviet Union, and Poland.[133]

On January 8, in a story primarily about the effect of the flu on New York hospitals, a small AP story was at the end, titled, "Flu Return Likely." The story originated out of Atlanta, and said that

> [t]he Hong Kong flu is on the wane in the United States, but it is likely to be around for several years, the National Communicable Disease Center reported today.
>
> However, a victim this year will probably be immune to the disease next winter when another, though milder, outbreak is likely, the center said.[134]

On February 8, the CDC reported in the *New York Times* that influenza activity had decreased in all but one state.[135] The next day, a feature article detailed the Hong Kong influenza outbreak in Hong Kong and how health officials there had responded.[136] The article framed "the race" between scientists and the virus as a fight against nature, reiterating a previous frame begun during this pandemic. On February 16, another feature story on influenza appeared:

> Scientists sometimes call it "original antigenic sin." It is not a new concept, but there is renewed interest in it today because it suggests a new strategy against an ancient enemy—the flu.[137]

The story, originating from Washington, chronicled the recent epidemic and past pandemics. It framed the virus and its antigens as a naturally occurring phenomenon for which immunologists were searching for a similar occurring vaccine that would have a broader application. The story essentially reiterated the tendency to frame this unknown phenomenon as an act of nature, as previous stories for this pandemic implied. Therefore, the burden of responsibility was transferred from humans, to scientists, to nature.

The last story in the *New York Times* for the pandemic period was on March 18, and described "a close relationship" between the Hong Kong flu virus and a flu virus that naturally infects horses.[138] Again, the framing suggested that influenza occurred naturally, but that it may be harbored or "recombined" in horses and pigs, which may give researchers an early starting point to isolate new subsequent viruses for vaccines.

Coverage in *The Times* (London) during the pandemic began October 1, with a story that expressed the framing of the Hong Kong flu to date. It said:

> The worrying feature at present is that the virus that has been isolated from patients during recent outbreaks of influenza in Hong Kong, Singapore, and Malaysia (A2/Hongkong/68, as it is known in laboratory jargon) differs from previous strains of the influenza virus A2 virus.
>
> In Britain, it is probable that the Hong Kong strain will be responsible for outbreaks of the disease this winter. Unfortunately, it differs so much from previous strains that few of us will have any residual protection against it.
>
> Equally worrying is the fact that the present influenza vaccine provides little protection against it, as has been demonstrated in Italy and Czechoslovakia. On the other hand, such vaccines do provide a modicum of protection and this, combined with the fact that those who have influenza in recent years may have a residue of antibodies to the new strain, suggests that the outbreak this winter should not be as severe as that of 1957.[139]

Therefore, the framing of influenza at the beginning of the flu season was one of cautious optimism. The next article indexed was not until November 5, 1968. The article, written by the medical correspondent, said

> [t]here are likely to be large-scale outbreaks of Hong Kong influenza between now and April, and until the necessary vaccines are readily available the best advice to sufferers is: Stay in bed until the temperature is normal.
>
> For most people the risk of complications is small. Available vaccine will go to the elderly and those with heart or lung disease until supplies become more plentiful.[140]

The framing of this story raised a little bit more of an alarm, and reiterated inoculation priority to high-risk patients. The last paragraph added to the alarmist frame:

> Supplies of the necessary vaccine are not likely to be available on a large scale before the end of this month and even then the quantity is not likely to be adequate for the demand.[141]

Toward the middle of November, stories appeared chronicling the demand for a vaccine before the epidemic. According to a pharmaceutical company:

> The demand for this new vaccine has been unprecedented. We have sold in a few days what we would normally sell in a year and orders are now subject to delay.
>
> Because of the short time available since the official identification of the new Hong Kong virus, the total output of the pharmaceutical industry would be sufficient for only a small proportion of the population.[142]

Several days later, the effects of this type of framing were expressed in a letter to the editor, which said:

> Sir,—In recent weeks there has been much publicity in the press concerning a so called Hong Kong influenza epidemic which is approaching these shores, and of a new vaccine which it is said to be readily available to counteract it. As a result of this many patients ask their doctors to immunize them with the vaccine. However, regular inquiries at one of the leading retail chemists in London have always brought forth the reply that there is no vaccine of this variety available and they do not know when there will be any.[143]

The sentiments of the writer expressed that there was frustration and anxiety because an epidemic was approaching and there was no available vaccine. He concluded the letter with a call for the Ministry of Health to handle a vaccination program rather than work with individual physicians.[144]

On December 10, 1968, an article in *The Times* (London) announced that the flu vaccine would be rationed by order of the Ministry of Health in order to deal with the shortage "caused by major breakdowns in commercial laboratories" in England.[145] The article explained that

> [d]rug companies have been instructed to give priority to supplying hospitals, general practitioners and wholesale and retail chemists so that medical staff and high risk patients can be vaccinated first.[146]

The framing of high-risk patients was similar to the 1957 epidemic, and the tone of the article suggested that the influenza narrative in the British press had now turned toward an alarmist one. A couple of days later, an article reported that the flu was expected in January or February 1969, and that only 400,000 vaccine doses had been distributed during November.[147] Thus, the alarm was heightened and the issue of a vaccine shortage was made more important. The article ended by chronicling the epidemic in the United States, and emphasized the severity of deaths by those infected with the Hong Kong flu.

On December 17, an article reported that the vaccine would not be made available in a timely manner because of "recent difficulties in meeting stringent requirements" to produce the vaccine.[148] Two days later, another article said, "Hong Kong influenza might reach Britain earlier than forecast," thus heightening the alarmist framing of a race for a vaccine and the anticipation of an impending epidemic.[149]

The next day an article on the front page reported that five people who had arrived from Canada and America were being tested to see if the illness they had come down with was the Hong Kong flu.[150] The day after, in another page-one story, it was reported that

> [g]rowing concern in Britain about the possibility of an epidemic of Hong Kong influenza was dismissed by medical experts last night. They said the concern was over "a non-existent situation."
>
> In the past few weeks there have been only about a half a dozen cases of Hong Kong influenza in Britain. The illness normally runs a mild course and some doctors think many people may have a natural resistance to it.[151]

The beginning of the article included a reprimand from government medical professionals that the public was worrying unnecessarily. However, the article ended with a discussion of what scientific experts had to say about the Hong Kong flu, which was contrary to what was said initially. This type of framing affirmed the alarm set off by the media, and did nothing to allay the public's perceived fears. A change in health policy was then announced, which stated that the general public would not have to fill out a "request for care" in the case that an actual epidemic occurred in England.[152]

At the beginning of the next year, on January 1, 1969, an article said that "British MPs" demanded "urgent government action to increase supplies of the vaccine developed to counter Hong Kong influenza."[153] This type of framing implied that there was extreme anxiety from the general public in wanting a vaccine for fear of the Hong Kong flu. On January 3, an article said that the British government could expect "a financial loss to the nation in excess of £400m," based on the Japanese experience of Hong Kong flu.[154] Not only was the general public framed as alarmed, but now the British government was too.

By January 10, 1969, when the flu and coverage were subsiding in America, Great Britain was beginning its epidemic.[155] The article explained a system devised by the British government to lessen the economic burden by appealing to "influenza victims to not go to their doctors unless they had chronic heart conditions or were bronchitics," and that

> influenza sufferers who take Mr. Ennal's advice and go to bed for a few days without bothering their doctors, have six days in which to obtain a medical certificate for payment of sickness benefit.[156]

Instead of raising an alarm or allaying fears, the article framed the government as actually giving incentives to influenza victims to not burden the health care system.

The next day *The Times* confirmed that the Hong Kong flu had spread to London.[157] At the end of the article was a brief message from the "Medical Correspondent" that said:

> Hong Kong influenza is not a serious type, and this outbreak will be similar to outbreaks experienced in previous years. The patient is affected for about two days. There can be a danger to the elderly, the very young, and people with chest complaints.[158]

While it appears that the medical correspondent might have been trying to calm the public's anxiety, he added a new group to the high-risk patient group, which was the very young. This might have actually done more harm than good and increased public fear, since this group had not been mentioned in any reports regarding the Hong Kong flu until then.

On January 20, the framing of influenza was altered contextually when a report of the outbreak was moved to the "In Brief" column.[159] The story was brief and merely said that four patients at a local hospital had been confirmed to be suffering from Hong Kong flu. This type of framing was, however, a return to previous coverage during the first two pandemics. In the same issue, a feature story entitled "Boo to 'flu'" presented a no-nonsense approach to influenza by saying, "It does not need a Minister of State to tell most of us that if we catch influenza the best treatment is bed, peace, and quiet."[160] The article implied that the framing of influenza had now switched to trying to calm any previous alarms.

The next day this trend was continued when a sizable story on page two reported, "Health experts wondered last night whether Hong Kong influenza might affect Britain less severely than was feared."[161] According to an official, the article said, influenza was impossible to predict. The rest of the article used statistics from the previous year to demonstrate that deaths were down and not up. This type of narrative was noticeably calmer and more optimistic than the coverage leading up to the epidemic. On January 28, another article reported that the "flu attack" had been mild so far.[162]

On February 4, however, a page-one story ran with the headline "Schoolboy dies from flu," and said, "Michael Day, aged 14, a pupil at Highgate Public School, London, died from influenza 30 minutes after arriving at his home."[163] Two days later a letter to the editor said:

> Sir,—I must repay the kindness of Highgate School and of scores of people (many of whom were unknown to my wife and me) by pointing out that the chances of Michael's sudden and unexpected death from influenza were infinitesimal. This is the tragedy.
>
> Yet your front-page report (February 4) made no attempt to present the occurrence in perspective and thereby implied a wholly unwarranted

> exaggeration of risk to other sufferers from this malady. My first duty is to put their minds at rest.[164]

This letter drew attention to how the framing of a story had a very definitive effect upon readers. The letter served to nullify the alarm originally raised in the initial story.

On February 7, a rather long feature by the medical correspondent ran under a large-font headline: "A case of fashionable 'flu'—or just a common cold?"[165] One would be hard-pressed to not get the gist of the article, which did indeed describe the difference between upper respiratory cold symptoms and the flu. A long history of the influenza virus with a description of the vaccine manufacturing process concluded the article. The framing of the article implied that perhaps some flu victims were actually suffering from a common cold.

The last two stories that ran during the defined influenza season were in the "In Brief" section of the newspaper. The first article, on February 8, said that

> some 13,000 cows are suffering from influenza in an epidemic which has spread from the Japanese northern island of Hokkaido, according to the Agriculture Ministry. About 50 cows have had to be killed.[166]

The second article said, "More than 2,258,000 people are reported to have been affected by an influenza epidemic in Poland," which was the same story picked up by the *New York Times*.[167] It was also interesting to note that while there was no influenza coverage carried in the final edition of *The Times* for the month of March 1969, this was the same time that the *New York Times* framed a severe influenza epidemic in London. One could imply that the British press decided no coverage was better than alarmist coverage.

COVERAGE AFTER THE PANDEMIC: APRIL 1969 THROUGH DECEMBER 1970

On May 31, 1969, the first story indexed after the 1968 epidemic in the *New York Times* was an editorial discussing the new preventative influenza drug introduced prior to the epidemic that had now been found to be of benefit to patients with Parkinson's disease.[168] A little over two weeks later another article about Symmetrel was reported which said that the drug had been beneficial to Russians suffering with the Hong Kong flu, contrary to American findings.[169] The debate surrounding the drug was not as important to the framing of influenza as was the fact that coverage had returned to that of framing research about influenza.

Four months later, at the beginning of the 1969 flu season, a story originating from the CDC in Atlanta reported that a major epidemic was not expected for this flu season.[170] Another story from the CDC announced that researchers were meeting at the CDC's headquarters to attend an international conference on Hong Kong influenza.[171] Then on December 15, 1969, a nonlocal story from London reported a "continental flu epidemic" was spreading across Britain, affecting "millions on the Continent."[172] The article also said that in Italy, "15 million were reported sick."[173]

Almost a week later, another nonlocal *New York Times* story from Geneva reported, "Virtually every country in Europe has been hit by Asian flu, and in several it has reached epidemic proportions, a report by the World Health Organization disclosed today."[174] While the framing of this influenza epidemic was alarmist, the article said that this epidemic was not the Hong Kong flu and was specifically referred to by the WHO as an Asian flu. The nonlocal coverage persisted, detailing outbreaks of a flu epidemic in Yugoslavia, London, and Rome.[175] Again, the epidemic in London received more coverage and more space in the *New York Times*.[176]

However, the next day an article by Lawrence Altman announced that the European epidemic was actually the Hong Kong flu.[177] The lead said:

> Throughout Europe and other widely scattered areas, epidemic Hong Kong influenza is sending millions of aching people to bed with fever and respiratory symptoms and causing thousands of deaths.[178]

Lawrence also attributed this information "from correspondents of the *New York Times*."[179] The rest of the article retold of the Hong Kong epidemic's path since it had been first reported in Hong Kong two years before. The article reiterated that United States experts did not expect to see a flu epidemic in the United States.

On January 31, 1970, the CDC reported new outbreaks of influenza along the East Coast states.[180] The article said that "in New York, outbreaks caused school closings."[181] On February 14, the CDC reported that "the Hong Kong flu is back," and forty-five states had reported influenza outbreaks.[182] While the CDC confirmed the cases were "the same as last year's," they said they did not expect these outbreaks to develop to epidemic levels.[183] A week later, the CDC reported that the flu in the United States had reached its peak level and was already declining.[184] There were no more stories indexed in the *New York Times* until November 19, when a story about the effectiveness of vitamin C as a preventative measure against colds and influenza was run.[185] The framing of influenza in the *New York Times* after the pandemic returned to previous trends established with the 1957 pandemic, which was to report on nonlocal epidemics and new research.

Coverage after the pandemic time frame in *The Times* (London) first appeared October 14, 1969, in an "In Brief" story that simply mentioned an influenza epidemic in New Guinea.[186] Several days later, again in the "In Brief" column another mention was made of the New Guinea epidemic, whose death toll had risen.[187] Then on October 22, a news story from a correspondent said, "At least 1,455 people have died of influenza in the highlands of Papua, New Guinea, in the past eight weeks."[188] The outbreak was reported to be under control and the Australian Army was flying in vaccines for New Guinea. While this nonlocal story did capture more attention than previous influenza coverage, a week later the epidemic returned to the "In Brief" column. This time the article only mentioned that scientists were investigating the epidemic in New Guinea.[189]

On November 1, 1969, the same story that ran in the *New York Times* ran in *The Times* (London), which was a story that originated from the "Nature-Times News Service" about the relationship of the influenza virus to animals.[190] Two weeks later, however, the New Guinea flu epidemic was expanded into a longer news story speculating upon which influenza virus had infected the island.[191] The nonlocal news coverage in *The Times* (London) carried a larger story telling of an epidemic that had struck "an estimated 13 million Italians."[192] The story said that local authorities had decided to accelerate "the process of supervising anti-influenza measures once the virus had been identified."[193] Several days later a story from Rome said that the flu epidemic was now in France.[194] Another report on December 19 said that Belgrade reported sixty deaths due to an influenza epidemic, and that influenza continued to spread quickly through Paris.[195]

The next day, on December 20, a political cartoon ran in the editorial section of the paper of a woman standing in the Ministry of Health's office, on the phone, saying, "No, dear, there doesn't seem to be anyone here to issue today's denial that there's a flu epidemic."[196] Up to this point, there had been no response from the British government in reference to the influenza outbreaks that seemed to be moving directly toward London. The cartoon literally illustrated this fact and created a framing device that the Ministry of Health was ignoring the potential epidemic. Two days later, the paper reported that the flu had struck London and was now interfering with daily business practices.[197] However, the framing of influenza was totally devoid of an official government response.

A week later a sarcastic editorial reiterated this frame and began with:

> The flashing of the red light for influenza once again is no cause for alarm. All the evidence to hand shows that the current outbreak is unlikely to be severe. The alert signaled by the hospitals in the Metropolitan and other areas merely means that they are taking sensible precaution of ensuring that as

> many beds as possible should be ready for the victims in the history of mankind.

It ended with:

> The otherwise healthy victim of influenza should simply take to his bed and stay there for a couple of days, dosing himself with hot drinks and whatever may be his pain-relieving favorite, whether it be aspirin or aspirin in some compound tablet such as can be obtained from any pharmacist. This will leave his family doctor free to cope with those of his patients for whom influenza may be a deadly hazard unless treated promptly.[198]

On December 30, an article identified the current flu epidemic virus in Britain as the Hong Kong flu of 1968.[199] In order to explain the lack of a response from public health authorities, the article said:

> Medical experts in Britain and Europe quietly predicted that it would soon reach them, and it did, via outbreaks in the southern hemisphere, in November. The speed of travel throughout the world makes it difficult for any country to avoid the infection. The World Health Organization, through its influenza centres, has followed its progress.[200]

While the article detailed the current influenza outbreak, it did so in a very nonchalant manner.

The next day a response to this article was printed in a letters to the editor section devoted entirely to influenza and entitled "This Winter's Strain of 'Flu: Not To Be Taken Lightly."[201] It read:

> Sir,—Whatever those who live in ivory towers may say, there is no doubt in my mind and many general practitioners that there is an influenza epidemic in many places.
>
> One of my former colleagues in London tells me of only two hours in bed in one night, and here in Salisbury things are very busy.
>
> What really distresses me is that the public are told it is a mild influenza. I have found this to be the understatement of 1969. In my experience it is a particularly severe form of influenza, requiring a minimum of one week off work and for most two weeks to recover from the debilitating effects. I would warn your readers to ignore all statements that it is mild and can be shaken off in a couple of days.[202]

Three other letters dealt with the effectiveness of vaccines, the spread of the disease, and the hospital bed system. For all the restraint that the newspaper demonstrated in not reporting about the influenza epidemic, the letters expressed an intense amount of anxiety felt by the public. Therefore, the alarm for a potentially severe influenza epidemic was framed through letters to the editor and editorials rather than through the responses of public health officials.

On January 1, 1970, an article attributed to the National Health Service said that the current epidemic was easing up.[203] However, the next day a large page-one story ran with a headline that said, "Flu deaths soar to 690 in week."[204] The byline read, "By Staff Reporters," and contained a comprehensive account of facts and figures surrounding the current epidemic. It led off with:

> Deaths from influenza in the week ended December 26 jumped to 690 from the previous week's total of 298, according to provisional figures released by the Department of Health last night. The final total will probably be slightly higher, the department said.[205]

Further down in the story, it said:

> Hardly any area of the country escaped the wave of absenteeism, with coal mines virtually at a standstill, all the major ports affected and large sectors of engineering and car industries badly under strength.[206]

This article demonstrated a return to the alarmist framing that had been established previously for influenza epidemics, but still lacked a medical arbiter response. A story the next day reported that sports activities had been affected by influenza, with many matches called off.[207] On January 7, another reported that while there had been a "brief lull" in the influenza outbreak in Birmingham, cases rose again to 240 having been admitted to hospitals.[208] Then, the next day, a page-one story reported that "influenza appears to be declining at last in London."[209]

On January 9, another page-one story ran the first story with a British medical authority attributed. The British Medical Association said, "This confirms the picture we had already built up from reports from family doctors all over the country that the outbreak was much more severe than was officially forecast."[210] The framing of influenza was now described by a medical arbiter as being worse than officials thought it would be, which might explain the lack of a response from medical officials early on.

By January 15, the red alert was once again lifted from London hospitals, as the number of deaths and the infected gradually declined.[211] A more sobering story two days later said that the influenza death toll for the last month was "nearly 7,000."[212] The article ended by saying that the death toll for the 1957 outbreak, which had been "previously regarded as Britain's worst," was 3,469.[213]

After the influenza epidemic subsided, coverage returned to influenza outbreaks in foreign cities under the "In Brief" column.[214] Another familiar frame returned after the pandemic during the remaining months of

1970, which was to highlight new research about cures, or previous influenza viruses.[215]

CONCLUSION

A new overall theme for the 1968 Hong Kong flu emerged. In addressing the social construction of disease and the response of public health policies, one could say that blaming nature for the pandemic emerged as the overall theme. However, in searching for a way to define the 1968 pandemic, a definition was reached almost immediately via scientific channels in naming the virus *scientifically*—A2/Hong Kong/68. Even though Hong Kong health officials tried to persuade authorities otherwise, the name stuck, because that is where and when the virus was actually identified scientifically. This reiterated the emphasis on the importance of science.

However, when it came to placing blame for the occurrence of the disease, instead of looking to the definition, or a foreign entity, a new frame evolved in the narrative discourse, which was to place blame on nature. In the framing of the 1968 disease, therefore, there was not much debate or framing devices used to actually define the disease. With a lack of argument, and acceptance that the virus was a naturally occurring event that man had not overcome, there were no new debates played out in the newsprint coverage. When humans are typically faced with unknown phenomenon, it is a natural tendency, historically, to place blame on nature.

The arbiters, whose evidence seemed not to be called to question, consisted primarily of scientists. There was a change in who was speaking on behalf of the United States, from the surgeon general in Washington to a spokesman in Atlanta at the CDC. This did not appear to be a result of media coverage, but was representative of the move to specialization in medicine, with specialists speaking on behalf of specific fields. Perhaps the most puzzling finding of this research was how the pandemic was covered by *The Times* (London). For the most part, medical authorities did not play any kind of arbiter role. When they did respond or were quoted, it was after the fact and not at the height of what seemed to be a time of heightened anxiety. If anything, editorials and the letters to the editor sections served as arbiters for this pandemic. This was a dramatic shift from previous coverage and deserves more attention in another study.

In reference to an underlying theme for this pandemic, the popularization of science resulted in a theme of faith in science, especially when scientists were, at the same time the pandemic was occurring, putting men into space and transplanting body parts successfully from the dead to the living. The narrative that had typically been fodder for science fiction had become a literal reality during the 1960s. However, rather than blame scientists, blame was assigned to nature. Both before and after the pandemic, coverage focused on new research, which was clearly representative of all coverage in the *New York Times*, *The Times* (London), and popular magazines.

Public health policies that changed were not overt, but when there was a relationship between coverage and policy, they did incorporate changes that resembled the 1957 pandemic. Specifically, policies changed to define a high-risk population that would receive priority vaccinations, to advocate inoculation prior to an outbreak, and to incorporate a better forecasting system via the WHO. The call for further research was also a new one, and tied in directly to the issue of blame. Clearly, the evolving mutating virus befuddled scientists.

NOTES

1. "Flu Epidemic in Soviet Cities," *New York Times*, 7 January 1967, p. 15.
2. "Russian Breaches Medical Secrecy," *New York Times*, 26 February 1967, p. 41.
3. A. Rosenfeld, "Breakthrough by Du Pont: A Drug That Blocks Viruses," *Life* 61 (10 February 1967): 60a–61.
4. Ibid.
5. "Influenza, Especially in East, Is Predicted for Next Winter," *New York Times*, 8 July 1967, p. 12.
6. Ibid.
7. Ibid.
8. Ibid.
9. Ibid.
10. "U.S. Medical Vacationers to Immunize Costa Ricans," *New York Times*, 29 July 1967, p. 25.
11. "Fast Centrifuges Give Purer Virus," *New York Times*, 29 July 1967, p. 27.
12. "New Clue Found to Spread of Flu," *New York Times*, 1 October 1967, p. 74.
13. L. M. Rhodes, "Killer on the Rampage: The Great Flu Epidemic," *Today's Health* 45: 24–27, October 1967.
14. R. D. Lyons, "Flu Season at Hand," *New York Times*, 8 October 1967, sec. 4, p. 6.
15. "Asian Flu Epidemic is Expected in East," *New York Times*, 20 October 1967, p. 41.
16. "Epidemic of Asian Flu Here Doubted by Health Official," *New York Times*, 9 November 1967, p. 52.
17. "City Aide Warns of Flu Epidemic," *New York Times*, 14 November 1967, p. 39.
18. Ibid.
19. W. Sulivan, "On the Archive Trail of the Causes of Disease," *New York Times*, 26 November 1967, sec. 4, p. 10.
20. H. M. Schmeck, "Influenza Season Begins Month Ahead of Schedule," *New York Times*, 21 December 1967, p. 25.
21. Ibid.

22. "Flu Outbreaks Spread in U.S.; Deaths Here Higher Than Usual," *New York Times*, 29 December 1967, p. 9.

23. "Flu Cases Fill London Wards," *New York Times*, 28 December 1967, p. 28.

24. See M. Tolchin, "Absenteeism Up in Flu Epidemic," *New York Times*, 4 January 1968, p. 13; "At Least 14 States Confirm Asian Flu," *New York Times*, 5 January 1968, p. 38; Val Adams, "Flu Curtails Attendance In Schools," *New York Times*, 6 January 1968, p. 31; and D. Bird, "City Deaths Rise with Flu Epidemic," *New York Times*, 11 January 1968, p. 1.

25. H. A. Rusk, "The Influenza Epidemic," *New York Times*, 7 January 1968, p. 60.

26. D. Bird, "City Flu Epidemic at Severe Stage," *New York Times*, 10 January 1968, p. 31.

27. "The Flu Strikes Again," *New York Times*, 12 January 1968, p. 26.

28. J. E. Brody, "Flu is in Season," *New York Times*, 14 January 1968, sec. 4, p. 10.

29. K. Teltsch, "Decline Predicted Soon in Flu Cases," *New York Times*, 16 January 1968, p. 77.

30. "City's Death Rate Dips First Time in Six Weeks," *New York Times*, 23 January 1968, p. 21.

31. Namely, Ibid.

32. "Flu Death Rate Dips in Most of the U.S.," *New York Times*, 3 February 1968, p. 29.

33. R. D. Lyons, "New Flu Vaccine Cuts Side Effects," *New York Times*, 28 February 1968, p. 18; and H. M. Schmick Jr., "Sprayed Vaccine for Flu Called Better Than Shots," *New York Times*, 6 May 1968, p. 49.

34. "Fiji Islanders Stricken," *New York Times*, 15 April 1968, p. 5.

35. "Flu Epidemic Doubted," *New York Times*, 7 July 1968, p. 36.

36. "Flu Alert in Philippines," *New York Times*, 1 September 1968, p. 25.

37. "Outbreak of Asian Flu is Expected This Fall," *New York Times*, 5 September 1968, p. 95.

38. J. E. Brody, "New Vaccine Speeded to Avert Epidemic in Winter," *New York Times*, 17 September 1968, p. 49.

39. Ibid.

40. Ibid.

41. Ibid.

42. J. E. Brody, "9 Cases of New Asian Flu are Reported in U.S.," *New York Times*, 27 September 1968, p. 9.

43. Ibid.

44. Ibid.

45. For the time period for this pandemic, 1967 through 1970, it was noted that *The Times* (London) had changed its format to one similar to the *New York Times*. Page one now contained news, rather than the classified section, as it had for the previous two pandemics.

46. "Warsaw," *The Times*, 16 January 1967, p. 8.

47. "New Influenza Strain Predicted," *The Times*, 20 January 1967, p. 7.

48. "Warsaw," *The Times*, 21 January 1967, p. 6.

49. "A doctor at the World Influenza Centre," *The Times*, 18 May 1967, p. 2.

50. "Two-day flu in South," *The Times*, 27 December 1967, p. 1.

51. Ibid.

52. "'Red alert' Sent to Hospitals," *The Times*, 28 December 1967, p. 1.
53. "'Flu' Virus Kills Five Babies," *The Times*, 29 December 1967, p. 1.
54. Ibid.
55. D. Jones, "Flu Epidemic Boost for Drug Profits," *The Times*, 29 December 1967, p. 17.
56. "Flu Epidemic Kills Two Babies," *The Times*, 30 December 1967, p. 2.
57. "Activities of Influenza Virus," *The Times*, 30 December 1967, p. 4.
58. Ibid.
59. "Influenza Red Alert to Stay," *The Times*, 2 January 1968, p. 2.
60. "Hospital Bed Demand Soars," *The Times*, 3 January 1968, p. 1.
61. "In Brief," *The Times*, 4 January 1968, p. 2.
62. "Rise in Brighton Death Rate," *The Times*, 5 January 1968, p. 2.
63. "Influenza Deaths 101 in Week," *The Times*, 6 January 1968, p. 3.
64. "Emergency Bed Demand Down," *The Times*, 10 January 1968, p. 2.
65. "Flu Hit Output in Engineering," *The Times*, 27 March 1968, p. 21.
66. "Asian Influenza Could Spread to Britain," *The Times*, 30 July 1968, p. 8.
67. "Influenza Stops Parliament," *The Times*, 9 August 1968, p. 1.
68. "Race to Find 'Flu Vaccine," *The Times*, 10 September 1968, p. 19.
69. "Epidemics Feared," *The Times*, 27 September 1968, p. 4.
70. H. M. Schmeck Jr., "An Antiflu Drug May be Tested," *New York Times*, 9 October 1968, p. 21.
71. H. M. Schmeck Jr., "F.D.A. Asks Maker of Flu Drug to Revise Claims," *New York Times*, 10 October 1968, p. 14. (The previous article was A. Rosenfeld, "Breakthrough by Du Pont: A Drug That Blocks Viruses," *Life* 61 (10 February 1967): 60a–61.)
72. "Few Deaths Laid to New Asian Flu," *New York Times*, 2 November 1968, p. 10.
73. "200,000 in Rome Have Flu," *New York Times*, 3 November 1968, p. 88.
74. Ibid.
75. "U. of Michigan is Testing a Flu Vaccine on Children," *New York Times*, 7 November 1968, p. 44.
76. "Hong Kong Flu Vaccine at End of Month," *New York Times*, 17 November 1968, p. 34.
77. "Vaccine Ready Soon for Hong Kong Flu; Outbreak Verified," *New York Times*, 19 November 1968, p. 93.
78. Ibid.
79. "First Flu Vaccine Shipped to Doctors," *New York Times*, 20 November 1968, p. 30.
80. Ibid.
81. See, "City Gets Set for Hong Kong Flu," *New York Times*, 23 November 1968, p. 49; "Prison in Colorado Hit by Flu Epidemic," *New York Times*, 24 November 1968, p. 62; and "Several Regions Report Further Outbreaks of Flu," *New York Times*, 1 December 1968, p. 67.
82. "Flu Kills 5 Aged in a Home," *New York Times*, 26 November 1968, p. 33.
83. "Apollo 8 Crew Gets Injections for Flu," *New York Times*, 4 December 1968, p. 95.
84. Ibid.
85. J. E. Brody, "Scattered Outbreaks of the Hong Kong Flu Occur Around City," *New York Times*, 5 December 1968, p. 40.

86. Ibid.
87. Ibid.
88. "Hong Kong Flu Now U.S. Epidemic," *New York Times*, 13 December 1968, p. 16.
89. Ibid.
90. "Flu Impact Grows Across The Nation," *New York Times*, 14 December 1968, p. 1.
91. "The Chameleon Virus," *New York Times*, 14 December 1968, p. 44.
92. "The Hong Kong Flu' Began in Red China," *New York Times*, 15 December 1968, p. 44.
93. Ibid.
94. G. B. Franklin, "Supply of Vaccine," *New York Times*, 17 December 1968, p. 46.
95. Ibid.
96. W. K. Stevens, "Northeast Especially Hard-Hit by Onslaught of Hong Kong Flu," *New York Times*, 17 December 1968, p. 95.
97. Ibid.
98. Ibid.
99. J. E. Brody, "City Giving 80,000 Hong Kong Flu Shots to Institutions Today," *New York Times*, 18 December 1968, p. 26.
100. Ibid.
101. Ibid.
102. M. Schumach, "City Attacks Flu as 200 Get Shots," *New York Times*, 19 December 1968, p. 1.
103. Ibid.
104. "The Flu Vaccine Shortage," *New York Times*, 19 December 1968, p. 46.
105. Ibid.
106. Ibid.
107. Ibid.
108. J. E. Brody, "O'Rourke Says Victims of Flu Face Complications From Cold," *New York Times*, 20 December 1968, p. 56; and A. H. Lubasch, "Fuel Deliveries Fall Short Here," *New York Times*, 25 December 1968, p. 1.
109. J. E. Brody, "O'Rourke Says Victims of Flu Face Complications From Cold," *New York Times*, 20 December 1968, p. 56.
110. M. T. Kaufman, "Death Rate Tops 1957 Flu Year," *New York Times*, 21 December 1968, p. 55; W. E. Farrell, "Office Absenteeism Up 50% Here in Flu Outbreak," *New York Times*, 22 December 1968, p. 27; J. E. Brody, "The Flu Virus is a Tricky Enemy," *New York Times*, 22 December 1968, sec. 4, p. 8; and "150,000 Flu Cases are Added to City," *New York Times*, 23 December 1968, p. 31.
111. J. E. Brody, "O'Rourke Says Victims of Flu Face Complications From Cold," *New York Times*, 20 December 1968, p. 56.
112. M. T. Kaufman, "Death Rate Tops 1957 Flu Year," *New York Times*, 21 December 1968, p. 55.
113. A. H. Lubasch, "Fuel Deliveries Fall Short Here," *New York Times*, 25 December 1968, p. 1.
114. Ibid.
115. M. Tolchin, "200,000 Heatless in 12? Weather; Flu Danger Seen," *New York Times*, 26 December 1968, p. 1.

116. D. Stetson, "All City Schools to Close 2 Days for Lack of Fuel," *New York Times*, 28 December 1968, p. 1.

117. Ibid.

118. E. Perlmuter, "Oil Crisis Abates but Flu Spreads," *New York Times*, 29 December 1968, p. 1.

119. Ibid.

120. V. Adams, "Blood Shortages Reduce Surgery," *New York Times*, 28 December 1968, p. 30; V. Adams, "Auto Injuries Add to Blood Demand," *New York Times*, 29 December 1968; E. Perlmuter, "City Doctors Give 10,000 Flu Shots," *New York Times*, 30 December 1968, p. 28; L. Fosburgh, "500 Here Answer Appeal for Blood," *New York Times*, 30 December 1968, p. 39; and D. Stetson, "Copter Delivers More Flu Vaccine," *New York Times*, 31 December 1968, p. 31.

121. E. E. Asbury, "'State of Peril' Continues Here,'" *New York Times*, 1 January 1969, p. 18.

122. Ibid.

123. "New Yorkers Give 200 Pints of Blood To Ease Shortage," *New York Times*, 2 January 1969, p. 64.

124. E. E. Ashbury, "City Flu Epidemic Continues to Ease," *New York Times*, 3 January 1969, p. 21.

125. "1st Heart Recipient of Year is Listed in Good Condition," *New York Times*, 3 January 1969, p. 21.

126. "Flu Deaths Reach 3,594 in 4 Weeks," *New York Times*, 4 January 1969, p. 25.

127. Ibid.

128. "Flu Toll Soared in Britain," *New York Times*, 5 January 1969, p. 76.

129. "City Ends State of Imminent Peril," *New York Times*, 7 January 1969, p. 42.

130. "W.H.O. Reports Flu is Reaching Europe," *New York Times*, 10 January 1969, p. 40.

131. Ibid.

132. Ibid.

133. "Flu threatens London Talks," *New York Times*, 12 January 1969, p. 74; "Moscow Flu Cases Double; Hong Kong Strain Identified," *New York Times*, 18 January 1969, p. 10; and "Flu Spreading in Poland," *New York Times*, 25 January 1969, p. 25.

134. "Flu Return Likely," *New York Times*, 8 January 1969, p. 35.

135. "Flu Cases Off in U.S.," *New York Times*, 8 February 1969, p. 28.

136. H. M. Schmeck Jr., "Hong Kong Flu: Story of the Close Race Between Man and the Virus," *New York Times*, 9 February 1969, p. 75.

137. "When 'Original Sin' Is Antigenic," *New York Times*, 15 February 1969, sec. 4, p. 6.

138. H. M. Schmeck Jr., "Asian Flu Linked to Equine Virus," *New York Times*, 18 March 1969, p. 14.

139. "Important Find in Treating Tumours," *The Times*, 1 October 1968, p. 5.

140. "'Stay in Bed' Influenza Advice," *The Times*, 4 November 1968, p. 3.

141. Ibid.

142. "Big Demand for 'Flu Vaccine," *The Times*, 11 November 1968, p. 19.

143. "Flu Vaccine," *The Times*, 14 November 1968, p. 11.

144. Ibid.

145. "Flu Vaccine is Rationed," *The Times*, 10 December 1968, p. 19.

146. Ibid.
147. "'Flu Epidemic Expected in New Year," *The Times*, 14 December 1968, p. 1.
148. "Influenza Vaccine Held up by Tests," *The Times*, 17 December 1968, p. 13.
149. "MP Fears Early Flu Epidemic," *The Times*, 19 December 1968, p. 3.
150. "Five Tested for Hong Kong 'Flu," *The Times*, 20 December 1968, p. 1.
151. "Immunity Hope as Flu Scare Grows," *The Times*, 21 December 1968, p. 1.
152. "Note May be Waived for Influenza," *The Times*, 27 December 1968, p. 1; and "Employers Welcome Flu Scheme," *The Times*, 28 December 1968, p. 9.
153. "MPs Demand on Flu Vaccine," *The Times*, 1 January 1969, p. 10.
154. "Cost of Flu 'Could be £400m,'" *The Times*, 3 January 1969, p. 2.
155. "11 Hong Kong Flu Cases in Midlands," *The Times*, 10 January 1969, p. 10.
156. Ibid.
157. "Hong Kong Flu has Reached London," *The Times*, 11 January 1969, p. 1.
158. Ibid.
159. "In Brief," *The Times*, 20 January 1969, p. 2.
160. "Boo to 'Flu," *The Times*, 20 January 1969, p. 5.
161. "Hong Kong 'Flu may not be Severe," *The Times*, 21 January 1969, p. 2.
162. "Flu Attack Mild—So Far," *The Times*, 28 January 1969, p. 6.
163. "Schoolboy Dies From Flu," *The Times*, 4 February 1969, p. 1.
164. B. Day, "A Schoolboy's Death," *The Times*, 6 February 1969, p. 9.
165. "A Case of Fashionable 'Flu—Or Just a Common Cold?" *The Times*, 7 February 1969, p. 11.
166. "In Brief," *The Times*, 8 February 1969, p. 5.
167. "In Brief," *The Times*, 13 February 1969, p. 6.
168. "Medical Serendipity," *New York Times*, 31 May 1969, p. 22.
169. "U.S. Flu Drug Gets Russian Approval," *New York Times*, 17 June 1969, p. 19.
170. "Experts Discount Major Epidemic of Flu This Year," *New York Times*, 3 October 1969, p. 20.
171. "Hong Kong Flu Parley Set," *New York Times*, 13 October 1969, p. 89.
172. "Continental Flu Epidemic Spreading Across Britain," *New York Times*, 15 December 1969, p. 14.
173. Ibid.
174. "Asian Flu Hits Europe," *New York Times*, 20 December 1969, p. 28.
175. "Flu Deaths Put at 190 in Yugoslav Epidemic," *New York Times*, 26 December 1969, p. 41; and "Jammed Hospitals in London Declare a Flu Emergency," *New York Times*, 28 December 1969, p. 21.
176. See "Flu Crisis Worsens in London as Disease Spreads in Europe," *New York Times*, 30 December 1969, p. 6; and "British Flu Toll 7,000," *New York Times*, 17 January 1970, p. 9.
177. L. K. Altman, "Hong Kong Flu is Affecting Millions in Wide Areas Around World," *New York Times*, 18 January 1970, p. 18.
178. Ibid.
179. Ibid.
180. "East Coast States Report Flu Cases," *New York Times*, 31 January 1970, p. 28.
181. Ibid.
182. "45 States Report the Hong Kong Flu," *New York Times*, 14 February 1970, p. 31.

183. Ibid.

184. "Flu Across Nation Reported at Peak," *New York Times*, 21 February 1970, p. 32.

185. "Vitamin C Called Cold Preventative," *New York Times*, 19 November 1970, p. 35.

186. "In Brief," *The Times*, 14 October 1969, p. 5.

187. "In Brief," *The Times*, 17 October 1969, p. 8.

188. "Outbreak of Flu Kills 1,455," *The Times*, 22 October 1969, p. 6.

189. "In Brief," *The Times*, 29, October 1969, p. 7.

190. "Did Asian 'Flu Start from Horses?" *The Times*, 1 November 1969, p. 3.

191. "Flu Threatens More Tribes," *The Times*, 15 November 1969, p. 4.

192. "13 Million Italians Hit by Influenza," *The Times*, 8 December 1969, p. 4.

193. Ibid.

194. "Flu Spreading in West Europe," *The Times*, 12 December 1969, p. 6.

195. "60 Dead in Influenza Epidemic," *The Times*, 19 December 1969, p. 5.

196. Illus. *The Times*, 20 December 1969, p. 8.

197. "Flu Holds up AA Service," *The Times*, 22 December 1969, p. 3.

198. "Down with the Flu," *The Times*, 29 December 1969, p. 7.

199. C. Warman, "A2 Flu Virus is a Seasoned Traveller," *The Times*, 31 December 1969, p. 6.

200. Ibid.

201. "This Winter's Strain of 'Flu: Not to be Taken Lightly," *The Times*, 31 December 1969, p. 7.

202. T. O'Keefe, "Letter," *The Times*, 31 December 1969, p. 7.

203. "Flu Showing Signs of Easing," *The Times*, 1 January 1970, p. 2.

204. "Flu Deaths Soar to 690 in Week," *The Times*, 2 January 1970, p. 1.

205. Ibid.

206. Ibid.

207. "Sport Cut by Influenza," *The Times*, 3 January 1970, p. 3.

208. "Birmingham Flu Rises," *The Times*, 7 January 1970, p. 4.

209. "It was Warmer in the Butcher's Fridge," *The Times*, 8 January 1970, p. 1.

210. "Gale-driven Oil from Sea Closes Town's Street," *The Times*, 9 January 1970, p. 1.

211. "Hospitals Normal," *The Times*, 15 January 1970, p. 2.

212. "7,000 Die from Flu in Month," *The Times*, 17 January 1970, p. 2.

213. Ibid.

214. See "In Brief," *The Times*, 3 February 1970, p. 8; 6 February 1970, p. 6; 12 May 1970, p. 10; and 24 June 1970, p. 6.

215. See P. Wright, "Hybrid may be Cause of Winter Flu," *The Times*, 12 May 1970, p. 10; "New Protection Against Influenza," *The Times*, 2 September 1970, p. 8; and "Pigs may be Spreading Influenza," *The Times*, 30 November 1970, p. 18. It is interesting to note that the last story in *The Times* (London) was a story about the potential link of pigs to influenza, especially when the next major news coverage of a potential influenza epidemic in 1977 referred to the vaccine as the swine flu vaccine.

Four

Media coverage of the three influenza pandemics told a story about an evolving public health threat, or battle, that still has not been solved or won. It is a continuing story. Each of the pandemics' newsprint coverage demonstrated a different narrative reaction to influenza via the framing devices. Therefore, the social construction of influenza did change over time. The 1918 Spanish influenza pandemic produced a narrative theme of intense anxiety and can be best described as a reactionary period. The 1957 Asian flu pandemic produced a narrative theme of scientific optimism, for which media stories presented a theme of control over disease by way of a vaccine and antibiotics. The 1968 Hong Kong flu pandemic theme used nature to explain the inability of scientists to control the disease, just holding it at bay via a vaccine. Together, the three case histories demonstrated that the social construction of influenza did change over time, and these changes were reflected in the narrative discourse, arbiter, and public health policy frames. A key thematic element across all pandemics was control, which was reflective of the ultimate goal for public health officials: to control and eradicate public health threats.

NARRATIVE CONSTRUCTION

Newspapers did not present abridged accounts of the pandemic, but presented information that fluctuated like the disease itself. Magazine coverage, on the other hand, was redundant and dated when compared to daily news stories. Magazines generally served to reiterate in a summarizing fashion what newspapers had already reported. However, the importance of including magazine coverage in this study was to demonstrate that the same information funneled out by newspapers was being distributed to a very large mass audience.

Previous studies of the 1918 pandemic referred to the pandemic as a "forgotten" epidemic. However, this was not the case, as demonstrated by the three different print media representations: national news, international news, and magazine coverage. A majority of the articles written about the 1957 or 1968 pandemics mentioned the 1918 pandemic. It was not forgotten, but retold, using similar war metaphors during the fifty years that this study spanned, both by reporters, editors, and in letters to the editors.

Newsprint coverage played an important role in socially constructing influenza. Narrative discourse for this analysis was defined as framing devices that initially defined the pandemic, the impact of influenza on the community, blame if it was present, and that war metaphors were used. A framing device for responsibility, or blame, for the disease was correlated with stereotypes, racial group, the victim's lifestyle, God or nature, or placing blame on government or medical institutions.

The Spanish Flu Pandemic of 1918

Narrative discourse for the Spanish influenza pandemic began with a definition in newsprint as a disease of concern for Germans and became a public health fiasco for the United States and the rest of the world. The coverage clearly demonstrated that influenza was a disease that was well known internationally. Several articles even made reference to a pandemic that occurred between 1890 and 1895. It had a defined history and was anticipated each year globally by citizens and public health authorities alike. However, as the death toll began to mount during 1918 and into 1919, a call for a response from public health authorities intensified. The disease frame changed from a typical case of the grippe, to a mystery disease of insurmountable cost to lives worldwide.

The Spanish influenza pandemic was first defined in newsprint as the German sickness. However, up to 1918, the disease was known as the "grippe" or "Spanish sickness." The first known documented identification, according to the coverage, told us that the disease originated in Spain, hence the Spanish sickness label. However, this was just a nickname and did not become a formal name for influenza until the severity of this particular flu strain was recognized. The naming of the 1918 flu, therefore, moved from a label of blame for a hated enemy of which many examples were given by the media, to a name that identified its place of origin. Therefore, the defining of the disease and initial blame for the disease used two framing devices that were collapsed upon each other.

Blame framing devices, while already identified as part of the social construction in naming the influenza pandemics, also evolved through the course of the pandemic coverage. Initially, the 1918 flu was blamed on

Germans, who were the enemy during World War I of the United States and Great Britain. Within the framing of blame, it was the German lifestyle that was used to explain the scourge and severity of the disease. Specifically, mediated stories reported that poor nutrition and a cold climate seemed to be the breeding ground for the infection. When it became apparent that the disease was spreading outside the ranks of the German army and into civilian populations, the German diet was blamed. When the disease spread out across the continent, poor nutrition due to the war-ravaged environment was blamed. When healthy Americans came down with the disease, there was a shift in blame to medical and government authorities. This shift brought about many debates in both the American press and British press and resulted in many public health policies, both formal and informal.

Another frame that developed during the course of naming the pandemics was to emphasize foreign or nonlocal influenza epidemics as being more severe elsewhere. This indirectly reinforced the blame framing devices by placing blame on a foreign, or nonlocal, city or country for the disease. This was another way to racially frame the blame for influenza. The most obvious instances of mediated coverage that framed this type of blame occurred when health authorities and media attempted to trace the infection route of the disease.

By the height of the pandemic, at the end of 1918 and the beginning of 1919, the name "Spanish influenza" became a permanent label for the 1918 pandemic. The narrative discourse for the 1918 flu changed daily in newsprint and represented a theme of not being in control. Public health authorities released death statistics, one day reporting a decrease in deaths, while numbers reported by hospitals or mortuaries would present conflicting information the following day, with an increase in deaths. Weekly death statistics were included with almost every story about the pandemic in the *New York Times*. Given the conflicting statistics and impact of deaths, media coverage reflected overly anxious reactions to the scourge of the disease.

The Asian Flu Pandemic of 1957

The narrative discourse raised by this pandemic was primarily a theme of optimism and faith in science. News stories rallied to miracle drugs, such as vaccines and antibiotics, and illustrated scientific advancements made since the last pandemic. While nonlocal coverage still tended to stay along the lines of the previous pandemic, this particular narrative frame practically diminished and focused instead on alerts, or local news. The threat of an epidemic affected the amount of print space devoted to debating how the local community would respond, emphasizing the impact of this pandemic. Clearly, scientific advances were framed within the context of the fifties, which reflected an intense amount of attention to anything scientific.

Additionally, in defining the 1957 flu pandemic, frames were drawn from the prevailing scientific notions of this time period. The 1957 pandemic was first called the "Far East" pandemic after its first documented appearance. During this time period, racial blame or profiling was used in reference to Cold War mentalities, which tended to place blame on Communist China and its citizens. Several stories pointed out that the virus could have been bred in unnatural conditions produced by the many refugees spilling out of China during this time period. The WHO, one of the first global health agencies, declared that the flu would be referred to as the Far East influenza. For the United States, the flu was named by the surgeon general's office in Washington as the "Asian influenza" epidemic. Therefore, in the United States the name "Asian" was used fairly consistently. British coverage, on the other hand, continued to call the 1957 flu by different names, varying between "Far East" and "Asian" influenza. Regardless, the Asian flu pandemic did not easily settle on a name, as did the 1918 pandemic.

From the onset of the Asian flu pandemic, all public health officials worldwide defined the emerging pandemic as mild, very contagious, but of no real health threat. This was primarily due to information from public health officials who implied that they were armed with new scientific weapons that could counter any attack by influenza. Officials often touted a vaccine to avoid the illness and new antibiotics to lessen the severity of the viruses' side effects such as bacterial infections and pneumonia. Consequently, the narrative discourse constructed a frame that focused on science as having a cure or at least control over the epidemic.

This optimistic narrative buckled, however, when the disease spread worldwide, and vaccines could not be produced quickly enough or in enough quantities to meet the public's demand. Coverage shifted from optimism in a scientific cure, to blaming health officials for not planning or timing the production of a vaccine appropriately. When it became apparent that public health officials had misjudged the situation, a new frame emerged to transfer blame for the deadly side effects from influenza to medical institutions that might be responsible for the creation of antibiotic-resistant bacteria found in hospitals. News stories appeared and suggested that even antibiotics might not be of benefit because of new antibiotic-resistant bacteria having been bred in hospitals. This served as a temporary distraction while public health officials scrambled to produce vaccines. By the time the frames split between the two controversies, the pandemic had begun to subside and resulted in another resurgence in faith in science because now there were more than enough vaccines to go around.

The Hong Kong Pandemic of 1968

Public health officials defined the Hong Kong flu pandemic immediately when it was given a scientific name for the actual location of the first isolated virus specimen—A2/Hong Kong/68. The name was an abbreviated version of the scientific name. Despite objections from Hong Kong health officials, the name was kept, reiterating the importance of science's role in public health and the now established trend to popularize anything scientific.

However, when it came to placing blame for the disease, instead of looking to the definition, or a foreign entity, the narrative discourse created a new frame, which was to focus on new research. That man had not conquered the flu virus was due in part to nature, the coverage explained, and therefore was a naturally occurring phenomenon. Like the Asian pandemic, the Hong Kong flu was also defined as mild, but might be avoided with the aid of science. The coverage reemphasized that the virus had not yet been conquered by science and, until then, it was an unwelcome visitor that one just simply had to put up with. With mediated stories lacking much argument, and with an acceptance that the flu virus was a natural occurrence, the narrative discourse focused on the potential for future research. Thus, a resulting theme of complacency, not control, emerged.

THE ARBITERS OF DISEASE

Sources and the type of information they provided created framing devices for pandemic influenza. Attention was paid to who was providing what information about influenza. As was anticipated, scientists, medical practitioners, and government authorities were used, and, with each pandemic, new arbiters were added. Additionally, news coverage itself changed, with few bylined stories during the 1918 pandemic, to an increasing amount of bylined stories by the end of the Hong Kong pandemic. The emergence of medical correspondents reflected the popularization of science. With each pandemic, as a frame shifted, there was also a shift in who was attributed, from individuals to health institutions, which also reflected the popularization of science.

The Spanish Influenza Pandemic of 1918

During the Spanish influenza pandemic, the arbiters in the *New York Times* consisted primarily of high-ranking public health officials preparing to do war with the disease. First, the New York City health commissioner was used regularly as a source for public health information and medical advice. The state health commissioner for New York did not garner as much attention as the city official, and, in several cases, it was the city official who was used as a source in stories originating outside of New York City. As the pandemic worsened, however, several other arbiters emerged, such as hospital administrators and port authority officials, whose responsibilities involved controlling quarantines for foreign vessels attempting to dock in U.S. ports. When the pandemic was on the verge of reaching epidemic proportions, the U.S. surgeon general began to emerge as a major source for information. If there was a conflict in information between a national or local spokesperson, newspaper editorials served as a mediating arbiter.

International coverage in the British news tended toward using politicians, physicians, and a medical correspondent as arbiters. However, information presented was very objective, while editorials and letters framed the issue at hand in a more subjective manner. During the 1918 pandemic in London, a new spokesman emerged in Britain in response to the influenza pandemic: the newly appointed minister of health. Prior to January 1920, Parliament determined public health care objectives and advised the public via the press.

The Asian Pandemic of 1957

With the advent of the Asian flu pandemic, arbiters increased significantly. They included public health officials, scientists, epidemiologists, insurance officials, and different specialized physicians. The World Health Organization generated advisories on a regular basis and released stories from Geneva, which were picked up by wire services. The influenza alerter system was an enhanced communication system enacted by the WHO that was supposed to open channels of communication between international, national, and local public health officials. However, this system was new and had not been completely accepted. An example of this was in the use of different names for the pandemic by different countries and their respective arbiters.

The Hong Kong Pandemic of 1968

During the Hong Kong pandemic, arbiters changed from individuals acting in their official capacity (1918 pandemic), to spokesmen and women acting on behalf of medical or government agencies and institutions (1957 pandemic), to the institutions themselves (1968 pandemic). The United States surgeon general was replaced by the Centers for Disease Control and Prevention's spokesperson. Stories were generated out of Atlanta instead of Washington. Instead of advice or information coming from general practitioners, now specialists dealing specifically with viruses were quoted. Pharmaceutical companies contributed significantly to the discourse about vaccines and future research, which in turn helped to reiterate the frame that all that could be done had been done, but new research was on the horizon. Arbiters also brought up previous pandemics to substantiate the naturally occurring phenomena aspect of influenza.

There were fewer editorials in the *New York Times* for this pandemic. However, the editorials and letters to the editor in *The Times* (London) actually served as the primary arbiters for the pandemic in England. While British public health officials acknowledged that they knew an epidemic was going to hit Great Britain, they did not react, nor did they issue any warnings. It was the editorials and letters that provided information and framed this pandemic.

PUBLIC HEALTH POLICIES

The impact on society that a particular disease had can also be ascertained by looking at policies that were created to deal with the disease. Public health policy frames, often represented by public health policies, consist of generally four types of options. They are defined by their approaches to preventative treatment or diagnoses and are: the medical approach, the behavioral approach, the ecological approach, and the future research approach to policy formation. The medical approach to public health policies consists primarily of identifying those at risk and then creating policies to treat them. The behavioral approach calls for changes in individual behavior and consists of policies that advocate how to avoid contracting the flu virus. The ecological approach for public health policies advocates changing the disease-promoting environment. This can range from quarantining international ports, to enforcing policies that affect a change in social or public meeting spaces. The final or fourth way that public health officials use to confront disease is a call for future research. Essentially, these approaches are reflective of the progress that public health officials made in eradicating a given disease or threat. If the disease has not been eradicated and health officials have acknowledged this, future research policies are perpetual, as long as there is a perceived threat. When the threat no longer exists, neither does the need for future research.

Public health policies could be formal laws or acts, or informal action in response to the disease. They could consist of courses of action as simple as a mediated message by health officials about how a hospital would manage patients, to a law with some sort of penalty to enforce a specific action. This was especially applicable to U.S. public health policy, where the system is not a national one. However, British public health policy differed because its medical system is socialized, and all manner of health policies reported were either discussed by Parliament (during the onset of the 1918 pandemic), or mandated by the Ministry of Health.

The Spanish Influenza Pandemic of 1918

The coverage demonstrated that, as the frame of influenza coverage changed, so, too, did public health policies. Public health policy moved from reactionary ecological measures to medical and behavioral measures. Additionally, a federal law was challenged as a result of influenza —Prohibition. In Great Britain, a Ministry of Health was created in 1919 in response to the framing of the Spanish influenza pandemic. On a global level, there were no policies or systems in place.

The predominant public health philosophy of the early twentieth century, as demonstrated by the 1918 pandemic flu coverage, was to react to the disease environment, rather than anticipate the disease. Initially, when word of the influenza epidemic was spreading, public health officials debated quarantines at all ports. When government officials reported that quarantining ports would disrupt the work of World War I, public meeting places were the next logical target for quarantines. However, instead of controlling or attempting to contain the spread of influenza, most cities, it was reported, simply canceled activities that would attract large crowds of people, including church services and school activities. Most of the ecological measures taken to try to contain the spread of influenza were generally after the infection or contamination had taken place.

When people began to get sick and death tolls mounted, public health officials turned to dealing with the care of those afflicted. This type of approach would be considered behavioral. Stories initiated by or attributed to public health officials called for citizens to live healthy lives, avoid stress, and get plenty of food and rest. Editorials called for citizens to stop congregating at dancing parlors and refrain from drinking too much liquor. Spitting ordinances and masks were then enforced by squads of sanitary police to help contain the spread of infection, all to no avail.

As the death toll continued to rise and cities were overcome with dealing with more corpses than coffins, some stories brought up the fact that a specific group of people were being affected by the disease—the young to middle-aged. This was the first time that a high-risk group was identified, but only in passing. Public health officials were too overwhelmed with the dead and were in the midst of the crisis before any action in reference to a medical approach could be taken.

Another interesting ecological public health policy that was enacted in New York City was to stagger work start times so that the subway system would not be congested with people. The system was actually hailed by the media as something that not only might have helped contain infection rates, but had a definite impact on the commuter system itself. However, when the crisis had passed, businesses returned to normal business hours.

Toward the end of the Spanish epidemic in the United States, when the death toll after the second wave in 1920 had begun to recede, a new frame emerged. Another issue was added to the influenza epidemic to its advantage, or so it appeared by way of the media-constructed stories. Prohibition was being enforced via the Volstead Act during 1920. Additionally, an old habit to use whiskey for medicinal purposes resurfaced during the influenza epidemic. Coincidentally, the greatest number of front-page stories in the *New York Times* focused on those influenza stories that included mention of the need for accessibility to whiskey for flu victims. The debate progressed to congressional hearings, which actually allowed for an amendment to the Volstead Act to permit the distribution of whiskey via a medical prescription. Once the amendment was in place and deaths had dropped off, the news essentially dropped off, too.

There were no more stories and never a call for future research. Public health officials simply did not have enough scientific information at that point to even know how to deal with the deadly virus. By the time they realized what was happening, it was too late.

The Asian Flu Pandemic of 1957

By the start of the Asian influenza pandemic, several scientific advancements had been made in the field of infectious diseases, such as the development of an influenza vaccine in the late 1940s and the development of antibiotics to ward off any deadly side effects from the flu. At the onset of the Asian flu epidemic, public health officials reported that they had no fear that there would be a repeat of the 1918 epidemic. After all, they said, they were armed with two lines of defense.

The narrative frames about the very scientific advancements that were at the foundation for the theme of optimism were challenged when officials could not support the narrative with actual policies. Public officials had the knowledge to produce a vaccine; they did not have the luxury of time. The first policy that was reported was by the U.S. surgeon general, who announced that the general public should be vaccinated, but that how this would happen would be handled on a local level. He did put forth a public service announcement via the media to make all physicians aware of how to diagnose and treat influenza victims. In this mediated bulletin, the surgeon general also put forth what he considered to be a priority list for who should be vaccinated first. Those determined to be in positions to take care of the general public or protect the nation and its cities were the basis for a working philosophy used in the policy formation of priority lists. The surgeon general told the American public that he would use the first batch of vaccines to inoculate the armed forces and then distribute vaccines by degrees of population and requests put forth by local public health officials.

This policy was an example of a preventative health policy whose focus was not medical or geared toward high-risk patients, but geared in an ecological approach. Essential workers chose a population that was most essential to the goings on of the nation's work or business. The policy did not take a medical approach in targeting the high-risk population identified in numerous media reports—the very young, chronically ill, and very old. Other countries, as reported by the media, interestingly enough, also picked up this policy.

By the start of the epidemic season in October 1958, stories reported that it was very unlikely that the general population could be vaccinated. Public health officials, it appeared, realized their predicament and switched from priority lists to transferring responsibility of who should be vaccinated to individual physicians. This was the same type of policy incorporated in Great Britain. Eventually, when the idea of a vaccine was futile, stories focused on framing a behavioral approach to public health policy by advocating that individuals learn to care for each other, rather than clog the health care system. This was especially evidenced by British coverage in *The Times* (London).

In an attempt to dissuade the general public from rioting for a vaccine, the effectiveness of vaccines was debated among public health officials and in editorials in U.S. coverage. Fearing that if and when individuals realized that there would not be enough vaccines to go around, antibiotic therapy and hospitalization were also debated. Several stories attributed by public health officials reported that the vaccine might not be a magic bullet cure after all, while other stories reported that antibiotics might be of benefit as a full-course treatment and that they did not work as a preventative treatment. Furthermore, it was reported that, if used as a preventative, antibiotics could induce antibiotic-resistant bacteria that would result in more deaths than the 1-percent death rate being reported for the Asian influenza epidemic.

While these debates were obvious frames in American media coverage, in the British press, they were undercurrents of the overall neutral frames. From the onset, British public health officials acknowledged that there would not be enough vaccines to go around and that, since the death rate was extremely low, citizens should go about their business and make the best of an unfortunate but normal situation, advocating a purely behavioral approach.

Toward the end of the Asian epidemic, officials also realized that the influenza infection time was quicker than the time it took for a vaccine to actually develop protective antibodies. New health policies ensued around the world in reference to just *who* would be considered a priority, given an insufficient supply and inability to produce enough vaccine in a short amount of time. What resulted, especially in America, was a new frame in public health philosophy, where consideration would eventually be given to those at medical risk over a physician's preferential choice, which was a medical approach to public health policy.

The Hong Kong Flu Pandemic of 1968

With the narrative discourse and arbiters placing blame on nature, a majority of the public health policies focused on the idea that more research would be key in dealing with influenza pandemics. Therefore, from the onset of the Hong Kong flu pandemic, public health officials advocated a neutral stance. Media reports did not represent panic, but were more objective and with much more scientific information.

The public health policies that did change were not overt, but incorporated changes hinted at during the 1957 pandemic. Public health officials moved from the idea of protecting essential workers or protecting the environment, to vaccinating the high-risk patient population first, which was a move toward a medical approach. Additionally, public health policies during this time period moved to advocating inoculation prior to an outbreak and to incorporating a better forecasting system via the WHO. Therefore, the approach taken at the onset of the Hong Kong flu pandemic was that of a medical one, with high-risk patient populations as a priority, but evolved into an ecological approach with an emphasis on future research.

Concluding remarks

Clearly, media coverage of the three flu pandemics demonstrated that there was a definitive change in the way influenza was constructed socially. The narrative started as a panicked out-of-control story during the 1918 pandemic. Then, in 1957, the narrative changed to an optimistic story chronicling an intense faith in science and then to a neutral narrative in 1968, where the future was portrayed as the crucial element in solving the mystery of the naturally occurring influenza virus.

The arbiters evolved as public health policies and health mechanisms evolved. During the 1918 pandemic, individual officials represented the majority of arbiters. During the 1957 Asian flu pandemic, new institutions such as the CDC and WHO entered the discourse, and, during the 1968 pandemic, with an ever-increasing number of medical specialists, public health was assigned official spokes-institutions rather than individual personalities.

Public health policies moved from panic-stricken actions that focused on the environment, to behavioral policies, and finally, to medical policies that actually focused on those most at risk or in need. The Hong Kong pandemic was representative of the level of cognitive sophistication that scientific advancement has brought, but was at the same time humbled by the fact that the virus had not been conquered. As reported by the media, the evolving mutating virus had befuddled scientists. However, since public health officials have not been able to produce a vaccine for the Spanish influenza virus of 1918, and they did not know the cycle of dormancy for the virus, future research for influenza is a perpetual policy because it is a continuing threat and a continuing story.

Recommendations for Future Research

However great the means of forecasting, diagnosing, and treating influenza, there is no conclusion or end to this particular disease. Therefore by studying and understanding how society has dealt with this disease, one can prepare for what will be either a continuing story, or a full-front battle with the disease. New mutated viruses and bacteria resistant to antibiotics continue to make themselves known. How society responds has been shown to influence public health policies, both in the United States and Great Britain. The theme for pandemic coverage moved from an unknowing panic reactionary public that produced many policies, to a common belief in the wonders of science with science-based policies, to finally the idea that influenza was a naturally occurring disease for which those most affected must be treated. The historical presentation of the media coverage and this framing analysis have demonstrated that public health policies are socially constructed systems which allow for self-correcting through the framing of the issues that define their very existence.

Since this text is essentially the first framing analysis to look at one disease over a significant period of time, there are many projects that could use this research as a starting place. One could address Spanish media coverage of the Spanish influenza pandemic in Spain, especially in reference to the narrative construction and how the pandemic was defined there. The same type of research could be done with Asian media coverage for the Asian pandemic of 1957 and with Japanese coverage of the Hong Kong pandemic of 1968.

This study serves as a methodological model to apply to other diseases and health issues, such as AIDS, organ donation and or transplantation, hepatitis, and actually any public health threat, as long as the study encompasses the first breaking story through a defined time frame to be significant.

The next logical chapter for this project would be to do a framing analysis of the 1977 swine flu vaccination program. One could question whether the frames established during the earlier pandemics were influential in the policy-making decisions during 1977. For the 1977 coverage, the National Newspaper Index could be used to focus on United States public health policy. Likewise, the fear of a pandemic in 1977 was worldwide: one could research whether or not the same was true for the United Kingdom.

In doing this study, this researcher has found that if one uses government documents, or medical journals, the indexed material correlating to a particular time period is not the same as the time period one is researching. For this study, public service announcements and bulletins covered by the media were often not published until several years after the event. Another consideration is that although *The Times* (London) has a very thorough index, the actual materials available on microfilm are not as complete. For those scholars who choose to use only the indexes as a source for discussion, or for a content analysis, be warned: many articles are cross-referenced under different subcategories under the initial keyword. In some cases, several different stories were listed under one indexed title. Therefore, relying on just the indexes for a research project is not advisable. What is advised is to evaluate all stories, rather than pulling a sample. As this text has illustrated, the 1918 pandemic has not been forgotten and was actually a reference point that framed and drove reactions to future pandemics.

Appendix A

Flu Pandemics	*Spanish Flu 1917–1920*	*Asian Flu 1956–1959*	*Hong Kong Flu 1967–1970*
No. of stories per season (Oct.–Mar.)	1918–1919 219	1957–1958 108	1968–1969 72
Year preceding	1917–0	1956–2	1967–16
Months preceding Jan.–Sept.	1918–47	1957–136	1968–27
Months after Apr.–Dec.	1919–36	1958–8	1969–9
Year after	1920–116*	1959–29	1970–10
Total number of stories for entire pandemic time frame for study	418	283	134 **Grand total:** 835

Source: *The New York Times Index*

Subject Keyword: "Influenza"

- For subject keyword by influenza name (Spanish, Asian, Hong Kong), all indexes referred or cross-referenced back to the initial keyword "influenza."
- Beginning with the second pandemic, the indexes indexed subject matter by year, instead of three-month intervals. The indexes did not use subindexing within the category. However, identifying information for each article varied from the notation of an illustration, chart, cartoon editorial, opinion piece, to a headline, summary blurb, or summarized list of information about the article.
- *There was actually a second wave of flu recorded for this time frame in the United States.

Appendix B

Flu Pandemics	*Spanish Flu 1917–1920*	*Asian Flu 1956–1959*	*Hong Kong Flu 1967–1970*
No. of stories per season (Oct.–Mar.)	1918–1919 148	1957–1958 75	1968–1969 32
Year preceding	1917–1	1956–9	1967–10
Months preceding Jan.–Sept.	1918–28	1957–143	1968–16
Months after Apr.–Dec.	1919–29	1958–7	1969–43
Year after	1920–13	1959–34	1970–26
Total number of stories for entire pandemic time frame for study	219	268	127 **Grand total:** 614

Source: *The Times Index* (London)

Subject Keyword: "Influenza"

- For subject keyword by influenza name (Spanish, Asian, Hong Kong), all indexes referred or cross-referenced back to the initial keyword "influenza."

Appendix C

Flu Pandemics	*Spanish Flu 1917–1920*	*Asian Flu 1956–1959*	*Hong Kong Flu 1967–1970*
No. of stories per season (Oct.–Mar.)	1918–1919 39	1957–1958 1	1968–1969 19
Year preceding	1917–0*	1956–2	1967–4
Months preceding Jan.–Sept.	1918–1	1957–3	1968–11
Months after Apr.–Dec.	1919–13	1958–2	1969–5
Year after	1920–11	1959–5	1970–5
Total number of stories for entire pandemic time frame for study	64	13	44 **Grand total:** 121

Source: *Readers' Guide to Periodical Literature*

Subject Keyword: "Influenza"

- For subject keyword by influenza name (Spanish, Asian, Hong Kong), all indexes referred or cross-referenced back to the initial keyword "influenza."
- Some 1918 magazine articles were listed under the 1919 index.
- *While there were no articles listed for 1917, in the index there were two articles listed for 1916 that were used for the influenza history to add more contextual information for the case study analysis.

References

Abelson, P. H. (1980). Scientific communication. *Science* 209: 60–62.

Albert, E. (1986). Illness and deviance: The response of the press to AIDS. In *The social dimensions of AIDS: Method and theory*, ed. D. A. Feldman and T. M. Johnson, 163–78, New York: Praeger.

Albrecht, L. J. 1992. A dose of information: What are your patients reading? *Texas Medicine* (Sept.): 36–42.

Alvarez, M., and R. Begue. 1999. *Eradication of infectious diseases: A goal for the next century*. Infectious Diseases Society of America, Thirty-seventh Annual Meeting, day 3, Nov. 20, 1999, http://www.medscape.com/medscape/cno/1999/IDSA/Story.cfm?story_id=912.

Angell, M. 1996. *Science on trial: The clash of medical evidence and the law in the breast implant case*. New York: W. W. Norton & Co.

Baker, A. J. 1986. The portrayal of AIDS in the media: An analysis of articles in the *New York Times*. In *The social dimensions of AIDS: Method and theory*, ed. D. A. Feldman and T. M. Johnson, 179–98, New York: Praeger.

Baran, S., and D. Davis. 1995. *Mass communication theory: Foundations ferment and future*. Belmont, CA: Wadsworth Publishing Co.

Barnard, C. N. 1972. Medicine and the mass media. *American Journal of Cardiology* 30: 579–80.

Basky, G. 1999. Media coverage of health stories often inaccurate, MDs report. *Canadian Medical Association Journal* 161 (4): 361.

Berger, M. 1951. *The story of the* New York Times*: 1851–1951*. New York: Simon & Schuster.

Berger, P. L., and T. Luckmann. 1966. *The social construction of reality: A treatise in the sociology of knowledge*. Garden City, NY: Doubleday.

Beveridge, W. I. B. 1977. *Influenza: The last great plague an unfinished story*. London: Heinemann.

Bird, S. E., and R. W. Dardenne. 1988. Myth, chronicle, and story: Exploring the narrative qualities of news. In *Media, Myths, and Narratives: Television and the Press*, ed. J. W. Carey, 67–86. Newbury Park, CA: Sage Press.

Blakely, D. E. 2001. *Mass Mediated Disease: A Case Study Analysis of News Reporting of Three Influenza Pandemics and Public Health Policy*. Hattiesburg: University of Southern Mississippi.

Blackmore, R. M., ed. 1975. *Cumulative Subject Index to the Public Affairs Information Service Bulletins, 1915–1975*. Arlington: Carrollton Press.

Boisaubin, E. V. 1988. Charity, the media, and limited medical resources. *Journal of the American Medical Association* 259 (9): 1375–76.

Bowman, J. S., and K. Hanaford. 1977. Mass media and the environment since Earth day. *Journalism Quarterly* 54 (1): 160–65.

Breo, D. L. 1989. Meet Vic Cohn—Dean of American science writers. *Journal of the American Medical Association* 262 (7): 968–70.

Brown, J., S. Chapman, and D. Lupton. 1996. Infinitesimal risk as public health crises: News media coverage of a doctor patient HIV contact tracing investigation. *Social Science Medicine* 43 (12): 1685–95.

Brown, J. D., and K. Walsh-Childers. 1994. Effects of media on personal and public health. In *Media effects: Advances in theory and research*, ed. J. Bryant and D. Zillmann, 389–416. Hillsdale, NJ: Lawrence Erlbaum Associates.

Burke, K. 1935. *Permanence and change: An anatomy of purpose* 1965 ed. Indianapolis: Bobbs-Merrill Company.

Burkett, W. 1986. *News reporting: Science, medicine, and high technology*. Ames: Iowa State University Press.

Cantor, N. F. 2001. *In the wake of the plague: The black death and the world it made*. New York: Free Press.

Cassedy, J. H. 1964. Muckraking and medicine: Samuel Hopkins Adams. *American Quarterly* 16 (1): 85–99.

Chesebro, J. W. 1984. The media reality: Epistemological functions of media in cultural systems. *Critical Studies in Mass Communication* 1 (2): 111–30.

Cirn, J. T. 1980. The birth throes of the Wisconsin Medical Practice Act: The physicians versus the newspaper editors. *Wisconsin Medical Journal* 79: 12–14.

Cole, B. J. 1975. Trends in science and conflict coverage in four metropolitan newspapers. *Journalism Quarterly* 52 (3): 465–71.

Coleman, W. 1974. Health and hygiene in the Encyclopedia: A medical doctrine for the bourgeoisie. *Journal of the History of Medicine* 29: 399–421.

Cormick, J. 1973. Medical advice in seventeenth-century journalism. *Journal of American Medical Association* 224 (1): 83–86.

Crosby, A. W. 1989. *America's Forgotten Pandemic: The Influenza of 1918*. New York: Cambridge University Press.

Croteau, D. 1999. Examining the "liberal media" claim: Journalists' view on politics, economic and social policy (including health care), and media coverage. *International Journal of Health Services* 29 (3): 627–55.

Cushman, P. 1982. Medicine at the turn of the century: Perspectives from the press. *New York State Journal of Medicine*: 81–84.

Davila, B. E. 1993. *La gripe Española. La pandemica de 1918–1919*. Madrid, Spain: Centro de Investigaciones Sociologicas (CSI).

Davis, R. J. 1993. Epidemiology on the agenda: The framing of chronic health risks by the news media (doctoral diss., Brandeis University, 1993). Dissertation Abstracts International, 54 (02): 9316011.

DeBakey, L. 1974. Medicine and the press: Resolving conflicts. *Clinical Research* 22: 214–25.

de Semir, V. 1996. What is newsworthy? *Lancet* 347: 1063–66.

Dunwoody, S. 1986. The scientist as source. In *Scientists and journalists: Reporting science as news*, ed. S. M. Friedman, S. Dunwoody, and C. L. Rogers, 3–16. New York: Free Press.

Dunwoody, S. 2001. Community structure and media risk coverage. *Risk* 15. Summer. http://www.fplc.edu/risk/vol15/summer/dunwoody.htm.

Dunwoody, S., and Ryan, M. 1985. Scientific barriers to the popularization of science in the mass media. *Journal of Communication* 35 (1): 26–42.

———. 1975. Academic and professional training patterns of science writers. *Journalism Quarterly* 52 (2): 239–90.

———. 1983. Public information persons as mediators between scientists and journalists. *Journalism Quarterly* 60 (4): 647–56.

———. 1987. The credible scientific source. *Journalism Quarterly* 64 (1): 21–27.

Dunwoody, S., and B. T. Scott. 1982. Scientists as mass media sources. *Journalism Quarterly* 59 (1): 52–59.

Emery, E., and M. Emery. 1988. *The press and America*, 6th edition. Englewood Cliffs, NJ: Prentice Hall.

Evans, W., and S. Priest. 1995. Science and social context. *Public Understanding of Science* 4: 327–40.

Fan, D. P. 1996. Impact of the mass media on calls to the CDC National AIDS hotline. *International Journal of Bio-Medical Computing* 41: 207–16.

Fine, B. 1933. *A giant of the press*. New York: Editor & Publisher Co.

Franklin, J. 1997. *The end of science writing*. The Alfred and Julia Hill Lecture, University of Tennessee, March 17, 1997. www.nasw.org/endsci.htm.

Freimuth, V. 1995. Mass media strategies and channels: A review of the use of media in breast and cervical cancers screening programs. *Wellness Perspectives* 11 (2): 79–107.

Freimuth, V. S., R. H. Greenburg, J. DeWitt, and R. M. Romano. 1984. Covering cancer: Newspapers and the public interest. *Journal of Communication* 34 (1): 62–73.

Friedman, S. M. 1986. The journalist's world. In *Scientists and journalists: Reporting science as news*, S. M. Friedman, S. Dunwoody, and C. L. Rogers, 17–41. New York: Free Press.

Friedman, S. M., S. Dunwoody, and C. L. Rogers, 1986. *Scientists and journalists: Reporting science as news*. New York: Free Press.

Friedman, S. M., S. Dunwoody, and C. L. Rogers, eds. 1999. *Communicating Uncertainty: Media Coverage of New and Controversial Science*. Mahwah, NJ: Erlbaum Associates.

Fulginiti, V. 2000. *The millennium in infectious diseases: Focus on the last century 1900–2000*. http://www.medscape.com/Medscape/GeneralMedicine/journal/2000/v02.n02/mgm0331.fulg/mgm0331.fulg-01.

Gellert, G. A., K. V. Higgins, R. M. Lowery, and R. M. Maxwell. 1994. A National survey of public health officers' interactions with the media. *Journal of the American Medical Association* 271 (16): 1285–89.

Glynn, C. J., and A. R. Tims. 1982. Sensationalism in science issues: A case study. *Journalism Quarterly* 59 (1): 126–31.

Goffman, E. 1986. *Frame analysis: An essay on the organization of experience*. Boston: Northeastern Press Edition.

Goldsmith, M. 1995. Directed to defend its *raison d'etre*, NIH holds communications conference. *Journal of the American Medical Association* 272 (10): 761–64.

Goodell, R. 1986. How to kill a controversy: The case of recombinant DNA. In *Scientists and journalists: Reporting science as news*, ed. S. M. Freidman, S. Dunwoody, and C. L. Rogers, 170–81. New York: Free Press.

Goodman, K. W. 1999. Philosophy as news: Bioethics, journalism and public policy. *Journal of Medicine and Philosophy* 24 (2): 181–99.

Gregory, R. 1991. Risk perceptions as substance and symbol. Pp. 1–10 in *Risky business: Communication of science, risk, and public safety*, ed. by L. Wilkins and P. Patterson. New York: Greenwood Press.

Hertog, J. K., J. R. Finnegan, and E. Kahn. 1994. Media coverage of AIDS, cancer, and sexually transmitted diseases: A test of the public arenas model. *Journalism Quarterly* 71 (2): 297–304.

Heuvel, J. V. 1991. *Untapped sources: America's newspaper archives and histories*. New York: Gannett Foundation Media Center.

Hillman, R. G. 1965. A Scientific study of mystery: The role of the medical and popular press in the Nancy-Salpetriere controversy. *Bulletin of the History of Medicine* 39: 163–82.

Hoehling, A. A. 1961. *The great epidemic*. Boston: Little, Brown and Co.

Horning, S., L. Walters, and J. Templin. 1991. Voices in the news: Newspaper coverage of Hurricane Hugo and the Loma Prieta earthquake. *Newspaper Research Journal* 12 (3): 32–45.

Houn, F., M. A. Bober, E. E. Huerta, S. D. Hursting, S. Lemon, and D. L. Weed. 1995. The association between alcohol and breast cancer: popular press coverage of research. *American Journal of Public Health* 85 (8): 1082–86.

Hume, J. 2000. The "forgotten" 1918 influenza epidemic and press portrayal of public anxiety. *Journalism and Mass Communication Quarterly* 77 (4): 898–915.

International Committee of Medical Journal Editors. 1993. Medical journals and the popular media. *The New England Journal of Medicine* 328 (17): 1283.

Jones, E. F., J. R. Beniger, and C. F. Westoff. 1980. Pill and IUD discontinuation in the United States, 1970–1975: The influence of the media. *Family Planning Perspectives* 12 (6): 293–300.

Kirkwood, W. G., and D. Brown. 1995. Public communication about the causes of disease: The rhetoric of responsibility. *Journal of Communication* 45 (1): 55–76.

Klaidman, S. 1991. *Health in the headlines: The stories behind the stories*. New York: Oxford University Press.

Kolata, G. 1999. *Flu: The story of the great influenza pandemic of 1918 and the search for the virus that caused it*. New York: Farrar, Straus & Giroux.

Kotulak, R. 1989. Sorting through the chaff. In *Health risks and the press: Perspectives on media coverage of risk assessment and health*, ed. M. Moore, 89–105. Washington, D.C.: Media Institute.

Kovarik, W. J. 1993–1994. *The ethyl controversy: The news media and the public health debate over leaded gasoline, 1924–1926* (Doctoral diss., University of Maryland–College Park, 1993–1994). *Dissertation abstracts international*, 55 (04): 9425070.

Kozloff, S. 1978. Narrative theory and television. In *Channels of Discourse, Reassembled*, 2nd ed., ed. R. C. Allen, 67–100. Chapel Hill: University of North Carolina Press.

Krieghbaum, H. 1959. Public interest in science news. *Science* 129: 1092–95.

Lane, D. S., A. P. Polednak, and M. A. Burg. 1989. The impact of media coverage of Nancy Reagan's experience on breast cancer screening. *American Journal of Public Health* 79 (11): 1551–52.

Logan, R. A. 1991. Popularization versus Secularization: Media Coverage of Health. Pp. 43–59 in *Risky Business: Communicating Issues of Science, Risk, and Public Policy*, ed. Lee Wilkins and Philip Patterson. New York: Greenwood Press.

Maccoby, N., and J. W. Farquhar. 1975. Communication for health: Unselling heart disease. *Journal of Communication* 25 (3): 114–26.

Maldonado, M. T., and Belsey, M. 1996. Culture, health, and the media. *World Health* (March–April): 28–29.

Mann, C. C. 1995. Press coverage: Leaving out the big picture. *Science* 269: 166.

Mannheim, K. 1936. *Ideology and utopia: An introduction to the sociology of knowledge*. New York: Harcourt, Brace and Co.

McCombs, M. 1994. News influence on our pictures of the world. In *Media effects: Advances in theory and research*, J. Bryant and D. Zillmann, 1–16. Hillsdale, NJ: Lawrence Erlbaum Associates.

McGee, D. E. 1996. Emerging meanings: Science, the media, and infectious diseases. *Journal of the American Medical Association* 276 (13): 1095–97.

McNeill, W. H. 1998. *Plagues and peoples*. New York: Anchor Books.

Miser, W. F. 1999. Critical appraisal of the literature. *Journal of American Board of Family Practice* 12 (4): 315–33.

Monto, A., D. Iacuzio, and J. La Montague. 1997. Pandemic influenza: Confronting a reemergent threat. *Journal of Infectious Diseases* 176 (Suppl. 1, 1997): S1–3.

Moore, M. 1989. *Health risks and the press: Perspectives on media coverage of risk assessment and health*. Washington, D.C.: Media Institute.

Nelkin, D. 1996. An uneasy relationship: The tensions between medicine and the media. *Lancet* 347 (9015): 1600–1603.

———. 1999. Foreword: Why is science writing so uncritical of science? *Risky business: Communication of science, risk, and public safety*, ed. by L. Wilkins and P. Patterson. New York: Greenwood Press.

Nuwer, D. L. S. 1996–1997. *The 1878 yellow fever epidemic in Mississippi* (Doctoral diss., University of Southern Mississippi, 1996–1997). *Dissertation abstracts international*, 58 (01): 9718190.

Oates, W. R. 1973. Social and ethical content in science coverage by newsmagazines. *Journalism Quarterly* 50 (4): 680–84.

Page, I. H. 1970. Science writers, physicians, and the public—Ménage à trois. *Annals of Internal Medicine* 73: 641–47.

Paisley, W. J. 1981. Public communication campaigns: The American experience. In *Public communication campaigns*, ed. R. E. Rice and W. J. Paisley, 15–40. Beverly Hills, CA: Sage.

Pan, Z., and G. Kosicki. 1993. Framing analysis: An approach to news discourse. *Political Communication* 10: 55–75.

Patterson, K. D. 1986. *Pandemic influenza, 1700–1900*. Totowa, NJ: Rowman & Littlefield.

Phillips, D. P., E. J. Kanter, B. Bednarczyk, and P. L. Tastad. 1991. Importance of the lay press in the transmission of medical knowledge to the scientific community. *New England Journal of Medicine* 325 (16): 1180–83.

Poe, A. 1999. Cancer prevention or drug promotion? Journalists mishandle the tamoxifen story. *International Journal of Health Services* 29 (3): 657–61.

Porter, K. A. 1936. *Pale horse, pale rider: three short novels*, 1998 ed. New York: Modern Library.

Priest, S. 2001. Cloning: a study in news production. *Public Understanding of Science* 10: 59–69.

Radford, T. 1996. Influence and power of the media. *Lancet* 347: 1533–35.

Ramsey, S. 1999. A benchmark study of elaboration and sourcing in science stories for eight American newspapers. *Journalism Quarterly* 76 (1): 87–98.

Rice, R. E., and C. Atkin. 1994. Principles of successful public communication campaigns. In *Media effects: Advances in theory and research*, ed. J. Bryant and D. Zillmann, 365–88. Hillsdale, NJ: Lawrence Erlbaum Associates.

Rich, J. T. 1981. A measure of comprehensiveness in newsmagazines science coverage. *Journalism Quarterly* 58 (2): 248–53.

Rosenfeld, A. 1999. The journalist's role in bioethics. *Journal of Medicine and Philosophy* 24 (2): 108–29.

Rosenkrantz, B. G. 1974. Cart before horse: Theory, practice and professional image in American public health, 1870–1920. *Journal of the History of Medicine* 29: 55–73.

Rubin, D., and V. Hendy. 1977. Swine influenza and the news media. *Annals of Internal Medicine* 87: 769–74.

Russell, C. 1986. The view from the national beat. In *Scientists and journalists: Reporting science as news*, ed. S. M. Friedman, S. Dunwoody, and C. L. Rogers, 81–94. New York: The Free Press.

Saliou, P. 1996. Crises communication in the event of a flu pandemic. *European Journal of Epidemiology* 10 (4): 514–17.

Satcher, D. 1994. Prescription: Communication. *Quill* 82 (9): 66–67.

Schneider, J. W., and P. Conrad. 1983. *Having epilepsy: The experience and control of illness*. Philadelphia: Temple University Press.

Schoenfeld, A. C. 1979. The press and NEPA: The case of the missing agenda. *Journalism Quarterly* 56 (3): 577–85.

Schramm, W. 1962. *Science and the public mind*. Institute for Communication Research, Stanford University (Issued for the AAAS).

Schudson, M. 1978. *Discovering the news: A social history of American newspapers*. New York: Basic Books.

Schultz, A. 1945. On multiple realities. *Philosophy and Phenomenological Research* 5: 533–75.

Schwitzer, G. 1992. Medicine in the media: The magical medical media tour. *Journal of the American Medical Association* 267 (14): 1969–71.

Shaw, D. L., and P. V. Nevel. 1967. The informative value of medical science news. *Journalism Quarterly* 44 (3): 548.

Shepherd, R. G. 1979. Science news of controversy: The case of marijuana. *Communication Monographs* 62: 1–36.

Shuchman, M., and M. S. Wilkes. 1997. Medical scientists and health news reporting: A case of miscommunication. *Annals of Internal Medicine* 126 (12): 976–82.

Singer, E., and P. M. Endreny. 2001. Reporting on risk: How the mass media portray accidents, diseases, disaster and other health hazards. *Risk: Issues in Health & Safety* 4, http://www.fplc.edu/medindx.htm.

Sofalvi, A. J. 1993. Mass media and the Inglefinger rule: Implications for health education. *Wellness Perspectives* 10 (1): 69–73.

Sontag, S. 1978. *Illness as metaphor*. New York: Farrar, Straus & Giroux.

———. 1989. *AIDS and its metaphors*. New York: Farrar, Straus & Giroux.

Spratt, M. 2002. Science, journalism and the construction of news: How print media framed the 1918 influenza pandemic. Paper presented at the annual meeting of AEJMC, Miami Beach, FL, 7 August.

Stacey, J. 1985. The press embargo: Friend or foe? *Journal of the American Medical Association* 254 (14): 1965–66.

Starr, P. 1982. *The social transformation of American medicine*. New York: Basic Books.

Steckler, A., J. P. Allegrante, D. Altman, R. Brown, J. N. Burdine, R. M. Goodman, and C. Jorgensen. 1995. Health education intervention strategies: Recommendations for future research. *Health Education Quarterly* 22 (3): 307–29.

Sumpter, R. S., and M. A. Braddock. 2002. Source use in a "news disaster" account: A content analysis of voter news service stories. *Journalism & Mass Communication Quarterly* 79, no. 3 (Autumn): 539–58.

Tannenbaum, P. H. 1963. Communication of science information. *Science* 140: 579–83.

Tuchman, G. 1978a. *Making news: A study in the construction of reality*. New York: Free Press.

———. 1978b. Professionalism as an agent of legitimation. *Journal of Communication* 28 (2): 106–13.

Turney, J. 1996. Public understanding of science. *Lancet* 347: 1087–90.

Turrow, J. 1996. Television entertainment and the U.S. health-care debate. *Lancet* 347: 1240–43.

Walters, L., and S. Hornig. 1993. Face in the news: Network television news coverage of Hurricane Hugo and the Loma Prieta earthquake. *Journal of Broadcasting and Electronic Media* 1: 219–32.

Warren, D. 1999. Daily news links you need to the information you need. *Health Progress* 80 (2): 12.

Watts, J. 1999. Media coverage of first transplantations fuels public distrust in Japan. *Lancet* 354 (9174): 229.

Willkins, L., and P. Patterson. 1999. *Risky business: Communication of science, risk, and public safety*. New York: Greenwood Press.

Winsten, J. A. 1985. Science and the media: The boundaries of truth. *Health Affairs* (Spring): 5–23.

———. 1994. Promoting designated drivers: The Harvard alcohol project. *American Journal of Preventive Medicine* 10 (3 suppl): 11–14.

Wolfle, D. 1980. Science: A memoir of the 1960s and 1970s. *Science* 209: 57–60.

Ziporyn, T. 1988. *Disease in the popular American press: The case of diphtheria, typhoid fever, and syphilis, 1870–1920*. New York: Greenwood Press.

INDEX

About the Author

Debra E. Blakely is Assistant Professor of Communication at the University of Houston–Clear Lake where she teaches media and public relations courses. She is also facilitating a national emergency preparedness communication program for Major League Baseball Security and Facility Management.